THE
HEALTHY FORMER ATHLETE

NUTRITION AND FITNESS ADVICE FOR THE TRANSITION FROM ELITE ATHLETE TO NORMAL HUMAN

LAUREN LINK, RD, CSSD

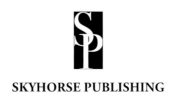

SKYHORSE PUBLISHING

Skyhorse Publishing books may be purchased in bulk at special discounts for sales promotion, corporate gifts, fund-raising, or educational purposes. Special editions can also be created to specifications. For details, contact the Special Sales Department, Skyhorse Publishing, 307 West 36th Street, 11th Floor, New York, NY 10018 or info@skyhorsepublishing.com.

Skyhorse® and Skyhorse Publishing® are registered trademarks of Skyhorse Publishing, Inc.®, a Delaware corporation.

Visit our website at www.skyhorsepublishing.com.

10 9 8 7 6 5 4 3 2 1

Library of Congress Cataloging-in-Publication Data is available on file.

Cover design by Tom Lau
Cover photo credit iStock

ISBN: 978-1-5107-3609-2
Ebook ISBN: 978-1-5107-3610-8

Printed in China

DEDICATION

I'd like to dedicate this book to my mom, Judy Kay Varnau, which is so clichéd, I know. The gesture is necessary for all the standard reasons: She got me involved in all kinds of sports growing up, everything from horseback riding to soccer, and she supported me in all of them, both financially and emotionally. From my early YMCA days through my college career, she missed only a single-digit number of games. Impressive. She's keeping that streak alive in my Normal Humanhood too. She's been at every Purdue Soccer Alumni Game since I've graduated . . . which is somewhat embarrassing, but she's earned it, I guess. More than all of that, I really owe my mom for making sure that I didn't grow up to be an excuse-maker. Nobody likes an excuse-maker. In fifth grade when I only made the B-team for basketball, there was no "woe is me" moment with discussions of how the coach must not have liked me or how the system is rigged. No, she said, "Well, they must have done something better than you, so figure out what that was and fix it!" No blaming the refs when we lost the big game. No, she said, "Well, you missed some opportunities on the field that could have won the game—focus on those." No excuses, just control what you can control. I considered thanking her for making endless spreadsheets based on my (and my team's) stats, which as a math major she literally couldn't help herself from doing . . . but those were annoying, and I stand by that. Thanks for everything else though, Judy K!

ACKNOWLEDGMENTS

First and foremost, I have to thank my sister, Julie Kartal, for support-ing the notion of this book from the very beginning and for agreeing to use her professional expertise to be my editor-in-chief. The latter might not sound like much when you consider that she has been an editor for several major news media outlets, but what if I told you that when she agreed to take this project on, she was living in France and raising four kids, including a 3-year-old and a 4-year-old? What if I also told you that at the same time, she was finishing her master's degree, working on selling the family business in France, and jumping through endless bureaucratic hoops to move her family back to America? Basically, she's a rock star. Thinking back on that process, I would also be remiss to not mention how thankful I am for Skype, Google Docs, and just technology in general.

I also have to thank Rachel Clark, most recently for being my mini content advisory board, but more so for being my mentor and guide in what I would absolutely consider my dream job. During my college days, teammates would ask me, "What do you want to do with your Dietetics degree?" and I would reply without hesitation, "I want to do what Rachel Clark does." (She was our sports dietitian and my academic adviser at the time.) Never would I have thought that I would end up back at Purdue quite literally doing what Rachel Clark does—first working under her, and eventually being passed the reins to become her successor as Director of Sports Nutrition for Purdue Athletics. I would also have never imagined that my professional idol would become a colleague and great friend. Rachel, I can say for certain that I would not be where I am professionally without your guidance, feedback, and occasional use of your hard-ass pants.

Lastly, I have to thank my fellow former-athlete husband, Logan Link, for listening with no complaints to my ideas about this book over the last few years, for waiting (almost) patiently to eat his dinner while I photographed our plates, and at times providing a male athlete perspective for various scenarios. I would also be remiss to not mention his handsome self being willing to participate in marketing photo shoots surrounding this project, conducted by our friend and graphic mastermind, Paul Sadler.

CONTENTS

INTRODUCTION

You've been setting your alarm clock for 5:30 a.m. for as long as you can remember. If not for an early weight-lifting session, then for 6 a.m. conditioning or to cram for a test you hadn't found time to prepare for between practices, team dinners, and rehabbing those nagging injuries.

It's an early wake-up call, but you love it. Live for it, really. You love the sense of camaraderie with your teammates, your best friends. You love that you're living your childhood dream.

Then one day you don't have to set that alarm anymore. It's a moment you always knew would come, but that doesn't make it any less gut wrenching. Your entire life has, in many ways, been devoted to your sport. When suddenly it's gone—or at least it feels sudden—it's like you're losing a part of yourself.

I've been there. In the fall of 2011, I finished my 5th and final season playing soccer at Purdue University, marking the end of my 18-plus-year stint as an athlete. Weird. It was one of the hardest things I'd ever had to deal with, a transition no one had prepared me for.

If you're reading this book, you've likely just finished your collegiate or professional athletic career (or soon will), joining the bruised and battered ranks of retired elite athletes. My goal is to help guide you smoothly through that transition.

In my first couple weeks of living this unfamiliar existence with no such guide to turn to, I took to blogging as a way to pass all my new-found time. The following is an excerpt from my first entry:

From the blog . . .

Officially Done

As a college athlete you live a completely different life than your average college student. A life full of lifting, fitness testing, early workouts, traveling to and from games, coaches and the need to constantly please those coaches, having to closely manage your time to get good grades, drug testing . . . the list goes on! Then, it all comes to a screeching halt and you're suddenly thrown into the real world, where time seems endless and your newly acquired lifestyle potentially leads straight to obesity. I figure this new lifestyle will bring all sorts of changes: some great, some sad, and hopefully none unhealthy . . . only time will tell.

A lot has changed since that first entry in 2011. I'm still a retired athlete, now enjoying my sport in a recreational league even though my joints still hurt way more than anyone's joints should in their mid-to-late twenties. But I'm now a Registered Dietitian and a Board Certified Sports Dietitian, working with elite athletes every single day.

What does that mean? It means I've been in your shoes, and I know how crazy hard the transition from athlete to Normal Human can be. I've also been in your pants (wait, what?), and with my professional expertise, I can help you manage this transition so those pants continue to fit. Maybe you'll even need to find pants a couple sizes smaller.

This book is designed to help you navigate the changes you're about to encounter. We'll discuss how to appropriately modify your diet based on Normal Human calorie expenditure, how to meal plan and grocery shop amid busy adult life, and how to save some money when it comes to food, so you have plenty of spending money for other fun adult things—like taxes and doctor appointments.

You'll learn how to approach working out in a way that doesn't involve a coach hanging over you and yelling out instructions. We'll even hit on the challenges you probably haven't considered yet—like forming an identity outside your sport and making friends since, ya know, you won't be constantly surrounded by teammates your own age who share your same interests anymore.

Throughout the book I'll also bring you more entries from my post-retirement blog to highlight some of the key issues you'll be facing and to illustrate some of my own mistakes with the hope that I can save you from making them. I've stopped blogging now that I've found plenty of ways to soak up all that free time that I enjoyed as a recent grad, but you can follow me on LinktoNutrition on Facebook, Instagram, and Twitter.

Normal Human* [noun]

A person who has chosen not to subject him/herself to countless hours of practice and conditioning, coaches with an affinity for shouting and inevitable joint pain early in life.

Example: I can't wait to enjoy life as a Normal Human after graduation.

*Disclaimer: The use of "Normal Human" in this book is intended to make a humorous distinction between your life as an elite athlete and your life after retirement. It is in no way intended to imply that you have not in every other way been a normal human in the traditional sense of the phrase.

1

BURNIN' THOSE CALS

From the blog . . .

So far, one of absolute best things about being a Normal Human instead of an athlete: You can work out for no other reason than "because I want to" . . . and I guess to stay healthy n' stuff.

Athletes spend most of their lives working out, especially in an endurance sport like soccer. You optimally want to stay fit throughout the year, especially when you get to college and there's the added pressure of having to make fitness tests constantly looming over you. All of these things make working out (which really can be an enjoyable thing) a huge burden. But not anymore, folks!

Recently a former teammate and I went on a run. A few miles in she asked if we could take a break because her knees were bothering her (don't get me started . . .). I gleefully replied, "Yes!! We *can* stop! Because we no longer have a need to build endurance, speed, or anything really!" This was a great revelation to both of us, one that I'm still smiling about.

Look for me around campus. . . . I'll be the one jogging slowly, then stopping to walk whenever I damn well please.

As if the transition to Normal Human isn't hard enough, the evolving framework of collegiate athletics has only made it harder.

While being pushed to your limits, you've also been pampered, fed, and provided coaching, clothing, medical care and everything in between. *(Division I athletes nod their heads, Division II and III athletes read on skeptically, thinking, "I guess some of that is true . . .")*

From a nutrition standpoint, a lot is about to change. Perhaps the biggest change is your calorie expenditure, or how much energy your body is burning each day.

As a college athlete, you were burning thousands of calories each and every day. Walking to class, weight lifting, conditioning, practice . . . all contributing to calorie expenditure much higher than that of your non-athlete counterparts.

As you approach retirement, you will probably fall into one of two groups:

The first group thinks, "I'll still work out just as much after I'm done playing my sport. After all, I *love* working out and I want to maintain my body composition!" This group is generally wrong. Get real, folks, it's called a job. Unless yours is working in a gym, it will suck your time and energy right out of your once-athletic body.

The second group thinks, "Psh. When I'm done with my sport, you won't be able to PAY me to get off the couch. I'm going to finally enjoy the R&R I never got before!" This group is generally closer to right—and usually regrets taking this stance.

Your goal is to find the middle ground between these two groups. In doing so, you should keep in mind the following:

10 REALITIES OF YOUR NEW LIFESTYLE

1. You'll realize it's nice to be able to take a more leisurely approach to your workouts. No coaches yelling, no predesigned workout templates . . . . While living a life of comparative luxury, you'll be burning fewer calories.

2. At this new leisurely pace, you'll realize you may need to spend a little longer at the gym than before to get the same results. But you're happy to do this, because you want to feel good in those jeans, baby!

3. You'll get a job. *(Hopefully. If not, maybe invest in a book on that as well.)*

4. Your job will take a lot of time and will probably involve more sitting than your previous lifestyle. Calorie expenditure will decrease further.

5. You'll wonder, "How did I previously fit all my workouts and practices into my busy schedule?" Then you'll remember that you had priority scheduling and a team of advisers working to make sure this happened.

6. Your job will make you tired. When you get home all you will want to do is sit. Maybe you'll muster up the energy to make dinner, or at least pick up the phone and dial for delivery. Sitting does not burn many calories—this is an important fact.

7. You'll realize sitting is nice. The more you sit, the more you don't want to get off your butt to work out. Calorie expenditure is at a new all-time low.

8. You will lose muscle. Sorry, but you will. (Don't panic—it's normal.)

9. Losing muscle can be frustrating. You'll wonder why the scale says you're about the same weight, but those jeans don't fit quite the same way as they used to.

10. This frustration may make you want ice cream or beer, both of which in excess can be unhealthy. Which will just bum you out more.

Sound over the top? Maybe a little, but you might be surprised. The good news is that there are ways to combat these changes. The reality is that you have to remain active in some capacity. What that activity ends up being is totally up to you, but remaining active is crucial to helping preserve muscle mass, promoting a healthy body weight, and generally making you a happier person because exercise produces endorphins n' stuff.

Current guidelines recommend that adults get 30 to 60 minutes of cardiovascular activity most days of the week. What, that's it? Sounds lame, but that's you now that you're a Normal Human.

In the process of deciding how you'll meet that activity requirement, you should start by locking down a few details. In the back of this book, you'll find several "Workout Plan" pages. This is a contract with yourself, so that you've put your commitment down in writing. I've provided lots of copies so that you can adjust your plan as you find out what works for you or as your needs change.

Go ahead and flip to the back and tear one out now so we can start putting your plan in place. You'll find that the last page of the book provides a couple of sample Workout Plans to reference as we go along. Once you've completed your plan, you should hang it on the fridge or somewhere you'll see it, or take a photo so it's with you on your phone.

STEP 1: SET YOUR BODY GOALS

The first thing you need to do in the Normal Human planning stages is to think about what your goals are surrounding your body weight and composition. Up until now it's likely that your sport required specific demands of your body. Maybe you've had to work to keep your body weight up or carry masses of extra muscle in order to be effective at your position or qualify for certain weight classes, and now that you're done you'd like to get down to a more natural weight for your frame. On the flip side, maybe you've had to be careful to keep your body weight down for similar reasons and would like to increase a little to a more realistic and casual weight for you. Or you may be focused on simply maintaining your current weight.

As a Normal Human, with no specific weigh-in or strength goals to meet for your sport, your goals should be centered more around body composition and what weight feels right for you.

Regardless of what your goals are, be realistic about them, especially as you feel out this new environment for the first time. If you are hoping to gain or lose weight, start with no more than 5- to 10-pound changes and never aim to gain or lose weight too quickly. You can always set new goals as you reach your old ones.

As we'll discuss later in chapter 2, never just quit lifting weights entirely, even if your goal is to lose muscle mass. By the same account, don't waltz into the weight room and try doing lifts that are drastically different than what you're used to if you're trying to gain muscle mass. Always ease into a new program or goal and adjust as you get a feel for it. In the back of the book you'll find tips on healthy weight gain (page 119) and healthy weight loss (page 123).

Have you decided what would be a realistic weight goal for Normal Human you? Write it down on your Workout Plan page now. As you work toward this goal, remember that the number on the scales is only an indicator of your progress. Your ultimate goal should reflect how you want to look and feel.

STEP 2: FIND A TIME

One of the most important things you need to do when evaluating your new workout plan is to determine when you will be able to fit your training into your schedule so that you will actually follow through with it. The most successful times for busy people tend to be early morning before work, during their lunch hour, or immediately after work—before they get home and decide that getting off the couch is the last thing they'd like to do. Decide what days and times you think will best fit your lifestyle and note them on your Workout Plan page.

As an athlete you were used to large time blocks set aside in your schedule to accommodate practice, lifting, and conditioning. With your new workout plan, one thing to keep in mind is that in this new reality you may only be able to find small blocks of time to work out. Don't be discouraged if you're only able to find 15- to 30-minute chunks of time—use that time to get a quick lift in or go for a walk or a run. Multiple smaller workouts can still be effective cumulatively. If you want to get your heart rate really pumping in a short amount of time, try running stairs, bumping up the pace of your run, or doing fast-paced calisthenics (body weight exercises like jumping jacks or push-ups).

STEP 3: FIND SOMEONE TO HOLD YOU ACCOUNTABLE

This won't be necessary for everyone, but if you have trouble motivating yourself (*you know who you are!*), seek out a coworker, neighbor or local friend, or family member who is willing to join you in your workout endeavors. Not only does this tend to make workouts more enjoyable (especially when you're still adjusting to not having your teammates around), but it's also much harder to leave someone hanging; thus, the accountability. Pull out your cell phone right now and browse your contact list for a possible workout buddy. Text them.

If you've moved to a new town and don't yet have a network of potential workout partners, this is also a great opportunity to meet people who share your interests. Post a message on the bulletin board at work or search Facebook for open activity groups in your community. Join the group and tell them you're coming to the next session/workout/run/lesson/match. You'll be more likely to follow through if they're expecting you.

If you're unable to find an interested partner or group or you really just prefer to go it alone, another option is to tell a friend or relative what your plan is and what your goals are. Sometimes that alone is enough to motivate you to follow through. If you're feeling really wild, post your goals on Facebook or Instagram. You've just ensured that your entire social network will be checking in to see how your new plan is going! Go ahead and write down how you'll hold yourself accountable on your Workout Plan.

STEP 4: DECIDE WHAT YOUR WORKOUT ENTAILS

Explore the opportunities in your community and be open to trying new activities. Make sure your plan includes both cardiovascular and muscle-building activities (we'll get to weight-lifting specifics in the next chapter). Here are a few places to start:

Hit the gym: Remember, gyms are more than just weight rooms. A membership at most gyms will buy you access to all kinds of equipment, a wide variety of group classes, and sometimes facilities such as swimming pools, climbing walls, and basketball or racquetball courts.

One important upfront consideration is cost. Working out in the real world can be expensive. Depending on where you live, you could be looking at $50/hour or more for a personal trainer and anywhere from $200–$1,000/year and up for commercial gym memberships. The good news is you have a job now! Budget early on for whichever activity you decide on. It might seem like a lot of money, but do you know what else costs a lot of money in the long run? Gaining unwanted weight. *(New, less flattering wardrobes, obesity-related health costs . . .)*

Seek out free trial opportunities to avoid wasting money on an activity or facility you don't like,* which can be discouraging and even lead to giving up an idea altogether. Many gyms run promotions offering a free trial week or trial classes. And if you have friends with gym memberships, they may have access to free guest passes to let you come with them and try it out.

Trying out group classes like yoga, Zumba, kickboxing, or CrossFit will give you a better feel for whether or not you want to work one of these activities into your plan. By trying new activities, you may find that working out can mean something much different than it did while

---

D-I athletes, prepare yourselves for disappointment. Most gyms, even the expensive ones, do not have facilities that can compare to the university facilities ~~you've been spoiled by~~ to which you've grown accustomed.

you were still competing in your sport. Diversifying your workouts can also help relieve nagging overuse injuries.

Friend alert: Group classes are also a great opportunity to meet people who share some of your interests. And for those single guys and gals—no better way to scope out some eye candy! Can you say bro tanks and yoga pants?

Most gyms also have personal trainers and possibly even nutrition professionals on staff, usually available to work with you at an additional cost. Tread carefully here and *always check credentials.* If you decide you want to consult with the nutrition professional at your gym, keep in mind that anyone can call him/herself a "nutritionist." However, you want to make sure you're working with a Registered Dietitian (RD or RDN). Similarly, you want to make sure that your trainer is NASM, ACE, NSCA, ISSA, or ACSM certified.

Also beware of any staff members at your gym trying to push supplements (vitamins, protein powder, etc.). It's not uncommon for these folks to earn part of their salary through product sales, so the supplement they're trying to sell you may be in their best interest, but not yours. Very rarely is any supplement necessary to see the results you want, as even the most elite athletes can meet their needs exclusively through food.

Find a new team: Maybe you're not quite feeling ready to give up the sport that you love. Depending on your sport, you may not have to! You may even want to try your hand at a new sport, or one that you haven't had time for since you were young.

If you're still on campus, most universities offer a large number of intramural sports, which provide a fantastic opportunity for staying fit and active as well as for making friends. If you've gone straight into the workplace, look for adult recreational leagues in your community. Go watch a game or two, and ask around to find out who you can talk to about getting on a team. Keep in mind these leagues generally involve a small fee.

Get outdoors: Are you reading this thinking, *The gym costs* how *much?!* Don't worry. There are plenty of things you can do for free, although some activities will still require a small cost upfront depending on what equipment you already have available.

Check out offerings at your local parks. Many cities are installing free outdoor exercise equipment as part of efforts to help their communities get fit. If yours hasn't, go old school. You'll be surprised at the workout you can get on monkey bars and jungle gyms. *(Maybe just avoid peak kiddie playtimes.)*

Benefits of Exercise Outdoors

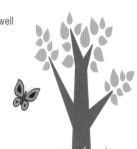

Vitamin D exposure
which promotes healthy bones and teeth and is preventative in nature for certain diseases.

Good for the mind
which can decrease instances of depression, anger, and tension compared to exercising indoors.

Good for the body
with natural factors like wind and hills creating increased exertion as well as a natural desire to push yourself harder.

Improved self-esteem
from a more private environment which can help build confidence.

Increased commitment
due to a generally happier demeanor for those exercising outdoors.

Cheaper than the gym
since many outdoor workout venues or trails don't involve a fee.

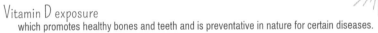

Free activities and about how many calories you can expect to burn

Activity (60 minutes)	Your Weight (in pounds)					
	130	155	180	205	255	285
Cooking	60	71	82	93	114	130
Cycling, leisurely	236	281	327	372	568	648
Cycling, moderate	472	563	654	745	795	907
Frisbee, leisurely	118	141	164	186	227	285
Gardening	236	281	327	372	412	455
General housework	148	176	225	326	284	324
Jogging (9-min mile pace)	649	774	889	1024	1135	1295
Jumping rope	600	740	880	1020	1166	1350
Light stretching/yoga	190	224	260	310	360	410
Push-mowing the lawn	325	387	449	512	583	639
Rollerblading	608	744	881	1017	1249	1425
Running stairs	768	915	1065	1210	1589	1813
Shooting hoops (alone)	207	242	287	326	397	453
Swimming laps, leisurely	413	493	572	651	712	789
Walking	195	232	270	307	350	397
Weight lifting, light	177	211	245	279	325	388

You'll notice this chart encompasses a wide range of different activities—some that rack up calorie expenditure very quickly and others that the former athlete in you may think could only count as "exercise" for local nursing home residents.

While calorie expenditure doesn't add up very quickly during activities like walking, stretching, and gardening, these contribute to your overall activity goals, so don't completely overlook them. On the other hand, it's best not to rely solely on those kinds of activities as you are unlikely to meet your energy expenditure needs without including more vigorous exercise.

Like many aspects of life we'll discuss, finding a balance of many different activities will help you stay invested in your plan and hopefully lead to a happier you.

STEP 5: GET OUT AND DO IT!

This is the most important step. Aim to include some sort of activity most days of the week. The more you can keep your energy expenditure

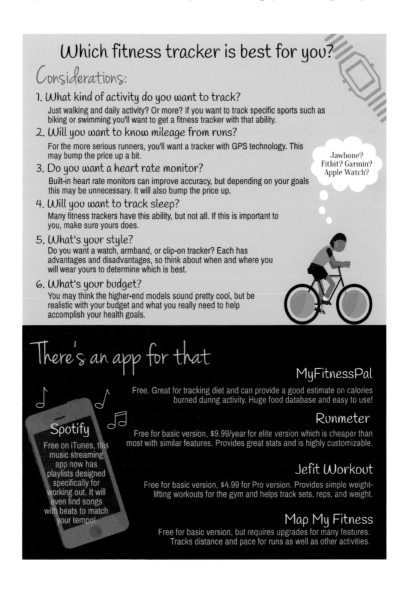

Which fitness tracker is best for you?

Considerations:

1. What kind of activity do you want to track?

Just walking and daily activity? Or more? If you want to track specific sports such as biking or swimming you'll want to get a fitness tracker with that ability.

2. Will you want to know mileage from runs?

For the more serious runners, you'll want a tracker with GPS technology. This may bump the price up a bit.

Jawbone? Fitbit? Garmin? Apple Watch?

3. Do you want a heart rate monitor?

Built-in heart rate monitors can improve accuracy, but depending on your goals this may be unnecessary. It will also bump the price up.

4. Will you want to track sleep?

Many fitness trackers have this ability, but not all. If this is important to you, make sure yours does.

5. What's your style?

Do you want a watch, armband, or clip-on tracker? Each has advantages and disadvantages, so think about when and where you will wear yours to determine which is best.

6. What's your budget?

You may think the higher-end models sound pretty cool, but be realistic with your budget and what you really need to help accomplish your health goals.

There's an app for that

MyFitnessPal

Free. Great for tracking diet and can provide a good estimate on calories burned during activity. Huge food database and easy to use!

Spotify

Free on iTunes, this music streaming app now has playlists designed specifically for working out. It will even find songs with beats to match your tempo!

Runmeter

Free for basic version, $9.99/year for elite version which is cheaper than most with similar features. Provides great stats and is highly customizable.

Jefit Workout

Free for basic version, $4.99 for Pro version. Provides simple weight-lifting workouts for the gym and helps track sets, reps, and weight.

Map My Fitness

Free for basic version, but requires upgrades for many features. Tracks distance and pace for runs as well as other activities.

up, the easier the transition to Normal Human will be, not to mention the healthier you will be. Besides, if it's an activity you enjoy you'll hopefully be happier too!

Think about whether you want to use a fitness tracking device and/or app to help keep you motivated and monitor your progress. These tools can estimate how many calories you burn throughout the day, how many steps you've walked, how restful your sleep was, and many allow you to track your food consumption too. This can be helpful in making sure you're meeting your goals, and many people find that they provide a fun way to hold themselves accountable by having contests with friends or coworkers. Proceed with caution when using these trackers around calorie recommendations. Many will underestimate your needs, especially if you select "weight loss" in the settings. Your calorie recommendation should be similar to what we'll calculate in Chapter 3.

Prices vary widely depending on features, from free apps to sophisticated smart watches that can cost several hundred dollars. There is a breakdown of the most popular styles on page 11.

STEP 6: BE READY TO ADJUST AS NEEDED

Even with a solid program in place, finding what works for you can be tricky. You may have a great plan and then have it ruined by a new job or other personal event in your life. Don't panic. Sit down and reevaluate your current workout plan and see what needs to be changed to keep you on track. Maybe it's a new workout time or new activity to adjust to the changing weather outside.

Whatever it is, take it in stride and remember, bumps in the road like these are common, and your former life as an athlete has prepared you well for them. Remember how much it sucked to show up for the first conditioning session after a month of not running? Same principle here, except there are no coaches breathing down your back to make sure it happens. Just make sure you address any problems early before you realize that months of inactivity have slipped by!

Common mistakes:

1. Be careful not to *overestimate* your energy expenditure. Even with a great workout plan, you are unlikely to burn as much energy as you did during your days as an athlete, when you had a coach pushing the pace and intensity of your workouts.

2. Avoid the "work out to eat" mentality. Too often people get in the habit of rewarding themselves for a hard workout by indulging in an extra treat. This will not help you reach your goals. Include these "fun foods" in moderation in your diet, but don't use them as a reward for following your exercise plan. By sticking to the plan with exercise AND diet, you will see your hard work pay off much more quickly.

3. Don't get too wrapped up in the numbers. Tracking your daily step count can be fun, but whether it's that or the number of calories you're consuming and burning, or your weight itself, don't let the numbers game turn into a true obsession as this can be a slippery slope leading to disordered eating/behaviors. Remember, your goal is to look *and feel* great and to stay fit and healthy.

4. Ultimately the goal is to be able to recalibrate and listen to your body without the external controls and numbers. If you're hungry, you should eat. When you're satisfied, it's time to move away from the table. After years of rigid schedules, now is the time to move toward trusting your body's cues and becoming more intuitive.

2

MUSCLE LOSS

This is where we make sure that your enjoyable activity plan not only helps use energy, but also addresses all that extra muscle you've packed on over the years. As a former athlete, starting to lose it is one of the biggest body shocks you'll face. It's unlikely that you'll have time to keep up the intense lifting regimen you had as an athlete, which means your muscle cells will start to shrink back to Normal Human size.

Besides being useful for things like moving heavy furniture or small cars, that muscle is important because it also burns a decent amount of calories even when you're just sitting around. So less muscle mass means you may need to consume fewer calories to maintain energy balance (more on that later).

For many male athletes, weight lifting is the easiest activity to continue in retirement. (*Gotta get swole, ya know?*) So, guys, you may not feel these effects as dramatically as female athletes, but keep in mind, you won't have a free trained professional writing your workouts for you anymore, nor will you have a facility that's specifically designed for that workout.

On the flip side, many female athletes, in particular, are eager to be done with their lifting regimen. As you will see from my blog post on the topic at the time, I fell into this group, and hardly touched a weight for the first few months of retirement (as you will also see, that was a bad choice):

From the blog . . .

The Downfall of PH

I red-shirted my freshman year. During the fall, the rest of the team had to take it easy when it came to lifting, to make sure they weren't too sore for games. Not the red-shirts! We lifted and we lifted and we lifted. When we weren't lifting, we were usually running a fitness test or playing against the people who showed up for the open tryouts (think jean shorts, scrunchies, and shin guards with ankle attachments). It was a glamorous life.

Through all that lifting I became quite strong and subsequently gained the nickname PH . . . for PowerHouse. I know, cute, right?

Much has changed since then. Recently I was working out and decided I would pump a little iron . . . gotta stay toned after all. Now I'm not crazy. I chose to do a set of bench press with 10-pound dumbbells. I could barely. Do. 10. Reps. What?! The girl who could squat 240 and clean 150 can barely bench 20 pounds?! This is ridiculous.

Since I really have no interest in trying to return to my PowerHouse self, I've accepted my new lack of strength. However, I have decided that it would be in my best interest to develop a strength training program that caters to my new Normal Human needs.

I will include exercises to improve the following functional activities (this is not an exhaustive list): opening jars, climbing stairs, getting out of beanbag chairs, pulling open heavy car doors, using multiple remotes at once, putting on skinny jeans, pushing things down to fit in drawers or suitcases . . . oh, how the great have fallen.

Okay, I was obviously being a little melodramatic, but I was truly shocked by how quickly I lost strength and noticed changes in my body! I went from thinking I'd never touch a weight again, to realizing I would have to find a way to work it into my routine.

Whether, as an athlete, you loved weights or hated them, you don't need to continue with the same routine. In fact, for most former athletes it makes more sense to modify your weight routine to better fit your new lifestyle.

Even though your routine might be modified, you'll want to make sure that you're still hitting all the major components of a good weight-lifting routine. A complete routine will hit:

BACK	**LEGS**
• Traps	• Quads
• Lats	• Hamstrings
	• Glutes
	• Calves
ARMS/CHEST	**ABS**
• Biceps	• Upper Abs
• Triceps	• Lower Abs
• Deltoids	• Obliques
• Pectorals	

If it helps, you can remember them by thinking, "If I don't hit all the core areas, I will turn into a BLAAb." That said, don't feel like you need to hit all of these muscle groups in every workout session.

Decide how many days per week you can dedicate to some sort of weight lifting—for most people 2 to 3 days per week is realistic—and make sure that you incorporate all of the muscle groups into your lifting schedule.

While 2 to 3 days per week is probably sufficient for those trying to maintain muscle size and tone, if your goal is to continue to build muscle or maintain a much larger frame, you may need to try to incorporate weight lifting into your schedule more often—closer to 4 to 5 days per week.

Most fitness professionals recommend that you group together exercises that fall into the same major muscle groups. For example, if you were able to lift weights two days a week, your schedule might look something like this:

Tuesday: Back and Arms/Chest
Thursday: Legs and Abs

Go ahead and write down on your Workout Plan which days you are going to fit in some sort of weight lifting.

It's also important to remember that these weight lifting sessions don't have to be an hour long anymore. In fact, depending on your goals, it is reasonable to assume you could get a weight session done in as little as 15 to 20 minutes once you've settled into your routine.

Make sure you pair it with at least 10 to 15 minutes of light cardio to warm up (such as riding a stationary bike, taking a brisk walk, or going on a light jog to the gym). And as always, you'll want to stretch before you get started. Remember, there won't be an athletic trainer ready and waiting to help you if you pull a muscle!

The final thing you need to consider before you hit the weights: What is your goal?

GOAL: MAINTAIN SIZE OR FURTHER BULK UP

Higher weight, lower reps

- Go as heavy as you safely can while still maintaining good form BUT never get under a bar without a spotter.
- Do 3 to 5 sets of each exercise, 5 to 8 reps each set.
- It may be worth your while to look into a gym membership. It will likely be hard to do everything you need to do at home.
- If you want to avoid the gym, look into purchasing an adjustable dumbbell set. These run anywhere from $150 to $300, which is cheaper than most traditional dumbbell sets. They're also much more compact.

• Remember my advice regarding supplements: Normally you can accomplish the same goal with food, even if that goal is to bulk up. Supplement companies heavily market to athletes trying to gain muscle, but supplements are poorly regulated by the FDA and in some cases they can be dangerous. Check out my post-workout recommendations on page 23.

GOAL: MAINTAIN MUSCLE MASS AND TONE, BUT DECREASE SIZE

Lower weight, higher reps

• Think light—using 5- or 10-pound dumbbells or even your body weight can be effective. The great thing about body weight exercises is that they're free!
• Do 2 to 3 sets of each exercise, 15 to 25 reps each set.
• There is also plenty of low-cost equipment that can be part of a great in-home routine:

Ankle/wrist weights: $15
Pair of dumbbells: $15
Resistance bands: $15
Medicine ball: $15
Stability ball: $10
Balance disc: $15
Pull-up bar: $25
Yoga mat: $20
Jump rope: $5
Stairs: $0 (Don't have any? Find a staircase outdoors, think *Rocky*!)

These are typical starting prices, though you can also easily spend $100 on a yoga mat or pull-up bar. Look online (try Google Shopping) or at discount stores such as T.J.Maxx for the best deals.

Athlete case files

Throughout this book I will bring you important lessons learned from the athletes I work with every day. Their names have all been changed to protect their privacy, but in this particular case file, I don't need to come up with an alias, because this cautionary tale comes from yours truly.

As established previously, I didn't lift much at all right after I finished playing soccer. But even once I realized that I needed to change that, I didn't go about it in the most balanced way at first, especially considering I have a dual degree in dietetics and health and fitness.

Like many soccer players, I always had pretty muscular legs. In particular, for whatever reason, I had very pronounced hamstrings. Genes maybe? A strong recessive hamstring gene? Now, before you Google "Lauren Link hamstrings"—I'm not talking freak show or anything, but they were sizeable.

After I started lifting again, I specifically didn't do any exercises that isolated my hamstrings, thinking that was a foolproof way to shrink them down to Normal Human hamstring size. Now, plenty of the exercises I was doing definitely work your hammies (lunges, squats, etc.) but while I was including exercises to isolate my quads, I was ignoring my poor hamstrings.

Long story short, my hamstrings, in all their glory, did NOT shrink. And in the meantime, I created a muscle imbalance that actually led to knee problems—like I needed any more of those! Once this was pointed out to me, I slowly started working to add hamstring exercises back into my routine, and lo and behold—some of those nagging knee pains went away.

The lesson? Even if you want to focus more on toning your muscles instead of growing them, don't ignore certain muscles or muscle groups. Especially ones that are used to getting a regular workout.

Who would have thought I could say hamstrings so many times on one page? Nine to be exact. Hamstrings. Now it's ten.

If you're feeling lost without your personalized training plan, there are websites such as www.acefitness.org/acefit/excercise-library that have extensive ad-free libraries with how-to videos of traditional muscle-building exercises:

There are also a number of online workout channels to give you inspiration and ideas for more original at-home workouts. Be ready for some of these to be chock-full of ads promoting various supplements and "burn away your belly fat" claims, not to mention questionable nutrition advice. In general, try to ignore everything that blinks and just stick to the workout videos:

blog.nasm.org/workout-plans

www.bodyrock.tv/workouts

www.mensfitness.com/training

www.fitnessblender.com/videos

www.befit.com/watch

www.nataliejillfitness.com/videos

A QUICK NOTE ABOUT BMI

BMI is a term that you (hopefully) didn't hear much as an athlete, but you may hear it in the future from doctors and other health professionals. BMI stands for Body Mass Index. It's a numerical representation of your height vs. your weight that health professionals sometimes use as a tool to measure a person's health and classify them into one of the following categories: underweight, normal weight, overweight, or obese.

BMI is not easily applicable to many athletes though. Because muscle weighs more than fat and elite athletes generally have a very high muscle mass, the BMI chart is unable to provide an accurate assessment. It's not at all uncommon for athletes to have a BMI that classifies them as overweight or obese, which of course isn't true.

This has two potential implications for the new Normal Human you:

1. If in the year or so following your retirement, you are told by a health professional that you are overweight or obese based on your BMI, don't immediately panic, especially if you've followed my advice and managed to stay in good shape. Explain your former elite athlete status and ask them to reevaluate their assessment taking your muscle mass into consideration.

2. On the other hand, as we've discussed, you're probably going to lose some muscle mass as a Normal Human. That means the older and more normal you get, the more frequently you may hear a doctor use this number to estimate your risk for chronic diseases. Just remember that BMI is only evaluating one thing—your height vs. your weight. It fails to consider countless other factors that may influence health.

You can find your approximate placement on the BMI chart on your own, but remember, it doesn't take into account your muscle mass:

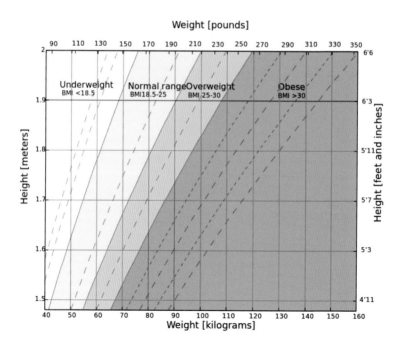

POST-WORKOUT RECOVERY

When I was an athlete, we rode our dinosaurs to practice and recovery with a healthy snack after practice was just starting to gain popularity. Nowadays, the importance of post-workout recovery to help restore energy levels, repair damaged muscle tissue, and promote maximal strength gains is widely accepted, and universities and professional teams everywhere provide post-workout options ranging from chocolate milk to fancy protein shakes and everything in between.

As a Normal Human, recovery is a good habit to keep, but as your workouts will likely be less intense, your post-workout snack should be smaller. If you're headed straight to lunch or dinner, that will cover your Normal Human post-workout needs.

A few questions I get asked frequently about post-workout recovery:

When do I need post-workout recovery?
After workouts of one hour or longer of moderate to high intensity.

How soon after working out do I need a recovery snack?
Aim for within 30-45 minutes of finishing your workout. And again, if you're going to be consuming a meal in that time frame, that meal can double as your recovery.

What should my recovery snack be?
For optimal recovery, aim to have a combination of carbohydrates, protein, and fluid, especially if you sweated heavily. See the chart below for recommendations.

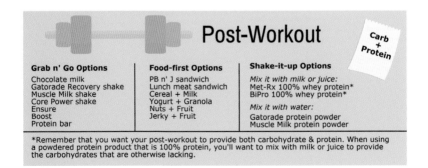

Post-Workout

Carb + Protein

Grab n' Go Options	Food-first Options	Shake-it-up Options
Chocolate milk	PB n' J sandwich	*Mix it with milk or juice:*
Gatorade Recovery shake	Lunch meat sandwich	Met-Rx 100% whey protein*
Muscle Milk shake	Cereal + Milk	BiPro 100% whey protein*
Core Power shake	Yogurt + Granola	
Ensure	Nuts + Fruit	*Mix it with water:*
Boost	Jerky + Fruit	Gatorade protein powder
Protein bar		Muscle Milk protein powder

*Remember that you want your post-workout to provide both carbohydrate & protein. When using a powdered protein product that is 100% protein, you'll want to mix with milk or juice to provide the carbohydrates that are otherwise lacking.

3

OH, THANKSGIVING . . .

From the blog . . .
Such a strange holiday. A time when we gather up our relatives, eat way too much, watch football games we probably don't care about, then wait in lines to spend money on things we don't really need (having spent the day discussing how thankful we are for the things we have) . . . all made possible by the Pilgrims, who took over the Native Americans' land and life as they knew it. Thanks, I guess? And sorry about our ancestors?

This was my first Normal Human Thanksgiving and after some deep intellectual thought I've come to the conclusion that this holiday certainly has things for which I'm thankful to be a Normal Human, as well as a few that make me wish I was still an athlete.

I'm thankful that I no longer have to worry about the fact that I didn't work out at all. It's a well-known fact that coaches love to run you into the ground after breaks, especially when they know you didn't even look at the workout packet they gave you. So, I'm very thankful to have no part in that anymore . . .

Now, on the other hand . . . while the post-break workouts were awful, they did force you back into shape pretty quickly. Since I no longer have that kick start to force me back into shape, my plan as of now is to strap my bags to myself pack-mule style and walk back to West Lafayette. Seems like a foolproof plan.

It should come as no surprise that your food intake is a huge aspect of the transition to Normal Human, and the one in which I, as a dietitian, am most interested.

Despite gobs of research showing how important nutrition is for optimal sports performance, many athletes still operate under the mantra of "I'm an athlete, so I can eat whatever I want." After all, you're burning thousands of calories a day, right? The fact that your performance probably could have been better if you had eaten better and not drunk like a sailor is now a moot point. So let's not dwell on that.

Let's dwell on the fact that you've now developed questionable nutrition habits that were probably only made worse by your extremely busy schedule, by the limitations of your Goodwill-salvaged kitchenware, and by loosened NCAA rules that meant your school could feed you pretty much around the clock. Then there's the likelihood that you've probably never really suffered any obvious repercussions of poor diet habits because you were burning those thousands of calories a day.

Even those of you who pride yourselves on eating well and who know your way around your kitchen undoubtedly still had to eat way more than a Normal Human just to keep up with calorie expenditure.

This means, for all of you, even with your workout plan in place, it's likely that you'll still have to modify your diet to some extent. In this chapter we'll talk about how to do just that, and in later chapters we will attack some scenarios that you will surely face as a Normal Human— like eating out, budgeting for groceries, packing a lunch for work, and cooking for yourself or your family.

We've talked about the importance of keeping your calorie expenditure up, so now let's talk about how many calories your body will need to meet your weight goals based on that expenditure.

First, we need to review a couple of basic realities:

If you eat more calories than you burn, you will gain weight.
If you burn more calories than you eat, you will lose weight.

This is an oversimplification of a very complex process, as the right number of calories for YOU depends on a lot of things. The good news is we can estimate it right now, so pull out your smartphone calculator.

STEP 1: CALCULATE YOUR BASAL METABOLIC RATE (BMR)

This is the amount of calories it takes your body to just do body-things like breathing, digesting food, and other necessary stuff.

To calculate yours, plug your information into the appropriate equation:

Women: BMR = 655 + (4.35 × your weight in pounds)
            + (4.7 × height in inches) − (4.7 × age in years)
Men: BMR = 66 + (6.23 × your weight in pounds)
            + (12.7 × height in inches) − (6.8 × age in years)

If you've done your math correctly, your answer should be a number in the low thousands, maybe in the ballpark of 1,400 to 1,800 calories per day for a woman or 1,800 to 2,400 calories per day for a man. Remember, this is *only* the number of calories your body needs to complete basic functions. See Step 2 to get an idea of total calories needed.

You can also use the online calculator at www.freebmrcalculator.com.

STEP 2: ACCOUNT FOR YOUR ENERGY EXPENDITURE

Take your BMR from Step 1 and multiply it by the appropriate activity factor listed below. This will give you an estimation of how many total calories you're currently burning on a day-to-day basis.

Sedentary (little or no exercise): BMR × 1.2

Lightly active (light exercise/sports 1–3 days/week): BMR × 1.375

Moderately active (moderate exercise/sports 3–5 days/week): BMR × 1.55

Very active (hard exercise/sports 6–7 days a week): BMR × 1.725

Extremely active (very hard exercise/sports and physical job or twice-daily training): BMR × 1.9

STEP 3: ALIGN YOUR CALORIC NEEDS WITH YOUR WEIGHT GOAL

In chapter 1, you set a realistic goal weight for yourself. This is the final calculation to set your calorie intake to a level that will help you reach that goal:

Want to *maintain* your weight? Great! You're done. If you consistently follow your exercise plan and aim for the calorie level above, you should be able to effectively maintain your weight.

Want to *lose* weight? You should take the number from step 2 and *subtract 300–500 calories*. If you consistently follow your exercise plan and aim for this many calories, this should help you lose weight at a safe and healthy rate of 1 to 2 pounds/week. If you lose any faster than that, it's possible that you're not adequately hydrating (hydration status can cause big swings in your weight). It's also more likely that you may be losing muscle, and remember, muscle is good. Check out tips for healthy weight loss on page 123.

Want to *gain* weight? You should take the number above and *add 500-1,000 calories*. If you consistently follow your exercise plan and consistently aim for this many calories, this should help you gain weight at a healthy and effective rate of 1 to 2 pounds/week. If you gain faster than that, it's more likely to be fat, as opposed to muscle. Check out tips for healthy weight gain on page 119.

Go ahead and fill in your daily calorie recommendation on your Workout Plan.

Before we move on to the next chapter where we'll discuss what you should be eating to meet those calorie goals, a quick rant about why being a dietitian can be so frustrating a few important things to keep in mind when it comes to where you get your information about diet and nutrition:

1. Everybody eats. Therefore, everybody thinks he/she is a nutrition expert. Shockingly, this logic is flawed. Case in point: I brush my teeth, yet I am not a dentist. I ride in planes, but I am not a pilot. I take medicine, yet I am not a doctor . . .

2. Change is hard, so when we hear non-nutrition experts spout off quick fixes, magic pills, and cure-all diets, they sound a lot more appealing than listening to a trained professional who will boringly tell us that it takes time and effort.

3. Non-nutrition experts = Dr. Oz, Oprah and 98 percent of the information found on the Internet. Also, a "nutritionist" is not a real thing. It requires no credentials to call yourself one. Before you take nutritional advice from someone, ask if they are a dietitian. If not, move on.

Bottom line: When it comes to diets, if it sounds too good to be true, involves cutting out an entire food group, limiting yourself to very few foods, or is only liquid, just don't do it. Glad I got that off my chest!

Athlete case files

While it's not necessary to count calories every single day, sometimes tracking your calorie intake for a few days can be helpful to get an accurate picture of what you're actually eating day to day. Now that you've calculated your daily calorie goal, it may be helpful to track your calorie intake for a few days to see how close you're coming to meeting your goal. It's not uncommon for people to be surprised that they're actually getting way more or less than they thought (usually more—those little nibbles throughout the day add up fast!)

Tracking calories is not necessarily an intuitive task for everyone, as I was reminded by Jordan. He and a few of his teammates asked me how many calories they needed to gain weight. Given that they were football players on our offensive line, they were already pretty big dudes. So to gain more weight during their heavy offseason training, I recommended that they probably needed somewhere between 6,000 and 7,000 calories a day. That's a *lot* of calories, but they were up for the challenge.

They started using MyFitnessPal to track everything they were eating. Only a day or two into this new adventure, Jordan came to me discouraged and said, "Lauren. There is no way I can eat 7,000 calories. I'm barely getting to 5,000 and I feel like I might actually explode." I was surprised because while 7,000 calories is a lot, Jordan was a big guy who loved to eat and we had talked about strategies to increase his calorie intake. Heck, though I would never need to, I feel confident that I could eat 7,000 calories in a day if I really tried. So I started looking through his food logs.

It didn't take long to identify the problem. Jordan was doing a great job of putting every single food that he ate into the app, but he wasn't accounting for serving size. Meaning, even though he had eaten three chicken breasts, he wasn't adjusting the serving size or the number of servings, so the app thought he had eaten only half of one chicken breast. I estimated that he may have actually been consuming close to 10,000 calories had he entered his meals properly. No wonder he felt stuffed!

4

WHAT TO EAT

Now that we've figured out an estimate of *how many* calories you'll need, it's important to talk about where those calories will come from.

In elementary school, you probably learned about the five food groups: grains, meat, dairy, fruits, and vegetables. When it comes to sports nutrition, we talk about food in reference to the three **macronutrients**: protein, carbohydrate, and fat.

With the exception of water and alcohol, every single food and drink that you consume will be made up of one of the macronutrients, or some combination of the three. Each of the macronutrients serves a purpose in our bodies and they are all important.

Popular fad diets often promote cutting out one entire macronutrient (like diets that promote little to no carbs). While these diets can promote weight loss, the problem is that they're usually not sustainable and people end up right back where they started—sometimes even heavier and feeling even worse. A balance of macronutrients is the way to go.

Balance is a concept that you'll hear me preach a lot. A balanced diet is immensely helpful when it comes to optimal athletic performance, but even now as a Normal Human, maintaining a balanced diet is more likely to provide a wide array of nutrients (to keep you healthy), help promote good body composition (to keep you looking good in those jeans), and it's just a lot more enjoyable to eat a variety of foods.

CARBOHYDRATES can be thought of as your body's fuel, with your muscles and your liver as the gas tank. When you eat carbohydrates, they are eventually broken down into glucose, a simple sugar (not the same as the white stuff you bake cookies with).

The body stores glucose a couple of different ways: The bulk of it gets stored as a molecule called glycogen in your liver and in your muscles, and a smaller amount stays in your bloodstream—usually referred to as blood sugar. These simple sugars are important because glycogen is responsible for a great deal of the energy production in your body, and your brain prefers to operate solely on glucose.

So what happens if you cut out carbohydrates (as promoted by many current fad diets)? Your body has to find something else to use for energy and brain power. It will burn some fat, but it will also tap into stored protein—in other words, it starts breaking down your muscle.

Losing muscle is never good, but in addition to that, people who aren't getting enough carbohydrates tend to drag a little. They're tired and might not be as mentally sharp as usual. This usually doesn't promote very productive workouts, nor does it make you a very useful employee!

On the flip side, many people eat more than enough carbohydrates. If you consistently consume more carbohydrates than you need, your body is more likely to store the extra energy as fat, and over a long period of time excess carb intake can make it harder for your body to digest sugar efficiently, which can lead to diseases like diabetes.

At the end of the day, it comes back to balance and choosing the *right sources* of carbohydrates. Foods that are rich in complex carbs also tend to be rich in iron and B vitamins, as well as fiber, which in addition to keeping us feeling full, helps promote healthy digestion and helps moderate blood sugar by avoiding extreme highs and lows.

Check out the chart on the next page for examples of nutrient-rich sources of carbohydrates. You'll notice that most are grains, especially whole grains. Whole grains mean that the entire grain from the plant is being used. A few common examples: whole-wheat bread or pasta, brown rice, and quinoa. Starchy vegetables such as corn, potatoes and peas are also very carbohydrate-rich, so even though they are indeed vegetables, we assign them to our carbohydrate group for this purpose. All fruit is very carbohydrate-rich, so when it comes to macronutrients, fruit falls into this group, but as we'll discuss in the next chapter, fruit has a special place on your plate so we'll leave it off this list.

Notice that you also don't see things like cake, cookies, or sweets here. These foods are indeed rich in carbohydrates, but mostly carbohydrates from added sugars so I've listed them here instead of including on our "everyday list."

It's also important that you're eating the right *amount* of carbohydrates. This tends to be the biggest mistake Normal Humans make when it comes to carbohydrates in their diet. Pasta, for instance, is not inherently bad, but think back to the last time you ate pasta—did you eat a small portion? Or did it cover your entire plate? For most of us, the answer would be the latter.

Additionally, we tend to eat multiple carbohydrate-rich foods together. Going back to the last time you ate pasta—did you start that meal off with breadsticks or garlic bread? These are perfect examples of overdoing it when it comes to carbs.

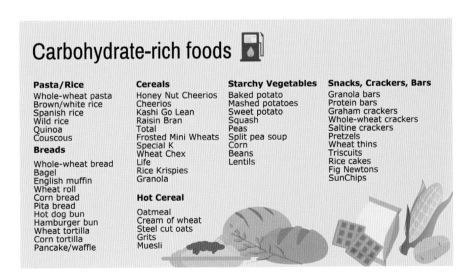

Carbohydrate-rich foods

Pasta/Rice
Whole-wheat pasta
Brown/white rice
Spanish rice
Wild rice
Quinoa
Couscous

Breads

Whole-wheat bread
Bagel
English muffin
Wheat roll
Corn bread
Pita bread
Hot dog bun
Hamburger bun
Wheat tortilla
Corn tortilla
Pancake/waffle

Cereals
Honey Nut Cheerios
Cheerios
Kashi Go Lean
Raisin Bran
Total
Frosted Mini Wheats
Special K
Wheat Chex
Life
Rice Krispies
Granola

Hot Cereal

Oatmeal
Cream of wheat
Steel cut oats
Grits
Muesli

Starchy Vegetables
Baked potato
Mashed potatoes
Sweet potato
Squash
Peas
Split pea soup
Corn
Beans
Lentils

Snacks, Crackers, Bars
Granola bars
Protein bars
Graham crackers
Whole-wheat crackers
Saltine crackers
Pretzels
Wheat thins
Triscuits
Rice cakes
Fig Newtons
SunChips

My advice: Try to think of carbohydrate-rich foods as a *side,* not the main course. A good reference can be your fist, which is about the size of 1 cup of cooked pasta or rice (*very tall basketball, football, and volleyball players, your fist may equate to slightly more, but your caloric needs are generally bigger too*). Aim to keep your portions of carbohydrate-rich foods about the size of your fist.

Athlete case files

I see and hear about fad diets all the time, most notably of late, the low-carb craze and the gluten-free fad. A male athlete called Brent came in to talk to me because he'd lost some weight and was feeling tired all the time. His training hadn't changed, but he was dragging in practices and feeling sleepy in class. I had him take me through what he eats on a normal day, and he started rattling off a list: eggs, sausage, peanut butter, lunch meat, cheese, burger patties with no bun, chicken, steak, veggies . . . it quickly became clear there was a theme here: no carbs. Brent confessed that he was indeed trying to eliminate carbs, because he saw a pro athlete doing it on Instagram. (*Cue heavy sigh.*)

I talked to Brent about the importance of carbohydrates not only for athletic performance, but also for energy in general. I explained that while there are a few situations that might warrant a low-carb diet, they did not apply to him, and that if someone is following a very low-carb or no-carb diet it should supervised by a doctor and/ or a dietitian. This is equally true of gluten-free diets. People who suffer from celiac disease must avoid gluten, but they represent a tiny portion of the population. The vast majority of people have nothing to gain by eliminating gluten, but they do risk creating nutritional deficiencies by cutting out important sources of vitamins, minerals, and fiber. Plus, gluten-free food is generally far more expensive!

It's possible that the pro athlete Brent admired was following a carb-free diet under the close supervision of medical professionals—but it's equally possible that he wasn't really following the diet at all, and that he was simply being paid to say he was. Which is the other important takeaway from Brent's case: Don't believe social media when it comes to diet and nutrition!

PROTEIN can be thought of as the body's building blocks. When you eat protein, it is broken down into different amino acids, which are then used to build new muscle, repair tissue, and keep all your biological processes running.

If you don't get enough protein, your body will struggle to build new muscle and the lack of certain amino acids can cause symptoms such as fatigue, muscle loss, and changes in your hair and nails.

Additionally, animal proteins are great sources of iron, and most protein sources are rich in B vitamins. Deficiencies of either of these can also lead to health consequences such as extreme

HOW MUCH PROTEIN DO *YOU* NEED?

Take your body weight in pounds and divide it by 2.2.

This number is your body weight in kilograms (kg). Take that number and multiply it by 0.8.

Now take your body weight in kg again and this time multiply it by 1.2.

This will give you a range to aim for in grams per day. If you're still highly active, you can go as high as 1.5 or 1.6 for your top-range multiplier. (*"Highly active" means similar to your days as an athlete . . . not that you walked your dog or went to Zumba today.*)

Example: If your weight is

154 lbs. ÷ 2.2 = 70 kg

70 kg. × 0.8 = 56

70 kg. × 1.2 = 84

So you would aim to consume between 56 and 84 grams of protein per day.

fatigue, nerve and gastrointestinal problems, and mental health issues like depression and memory loss.

Nevertheless, American diets rarely lack sufficient protein. As an athlete you needed quite a bit more protein than most average adults. Now that you're a Normal Human, you'll need considerably less—even if you remain pretty active. In fact, especially given how oversized portions tend to be, most adults get well over the recommended daily amount, which is only around 60–70 grams per day.

Consuming too much protein, especially from sources high in fat, can also cause its fair share of problems, including high cholesterol. And keep in mind, your body can only use about 20–30 grams of protein toward muscle synthesis at one time. So, eating more protein (or taking large amounts of amino acid supplements) does NOT necessarily equal more muscle.

Again, healthy protein consumption comes down to balance. It's much healthier and more effective to include smaller amounts (20–30 grams) of protein consistently throughout the day because it's broken down relatively slowly in your stomach and can help you to stay full longer. Eating smaller amounts also helps promote optimal protein synthesis.

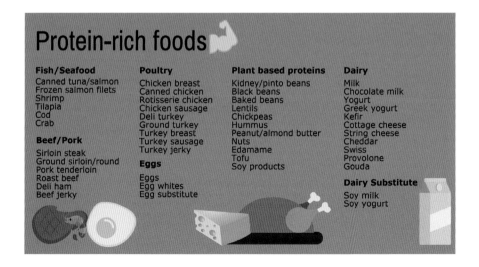

Protein-rich foods

Fish/Seafood
Canned tuna/salmon
Frozen salmon filets
Shrimp
Tilapia
Cod
Crab

Beef/Pork
Sirloin steak
Ground sirloin/round
Pork tenderloin
Roast beef
Deli ham
Beef jerky

Poultry
Chicken breast
Canned chicken
Rotisserie chicken
Chicken sausage
Deli turkey
Ground turkey
Turkey breast
Turkey sausage
Turkey jerky

Eggs
Eggs
Egg whites
Egg substitute

Plant based proteins
Kidney/pinto beans
Black beans
Baked beans
Lentils
Chickpeas
Hummus
Peanut/almond butter
Nuts
Edamame
Tofu
Soy products

Dairy
Milk
Chocolate milk
Yogurt
Greek yogurt
Kefir
Cottage cheese
String cheese
Cheddar
Swiss
Provolone
Gouda

Dairy Substitute
Soy milk
Soy yogurt

Just as there are healthy and less healthy carbohydrate sources, there are healthy protein sources and less healthy protein sources. All of them can have a place in your diet, but you should be eating mostly lean proteins. Check out the protein-rich foods chart for a list of nice lean protein options. Note that you won't find bacon, sausage, or other highly processed meats on this list. Just like the carbohydrates that were largely processed sugars, these processed protein options are higher in unhealthy fats and additives and are best eaten in moderation.

One final note on protein for those of you who are **vegetarian or vegan**. If you're not eating any meat or animal-derived foods, you're going to need to put more effort toward getting adequate protein each day from nonmeat sources such as nuts and seeds, nut butters, beans, legumes, whole grains, and tofu and other soy products. Vegetarians can also include eggs and dairy products. Many vegetarians and vegans will need to supplement with B vitamins, specifically B_{12}, to avoid deficiencies. Consult with your doctor or dietitian to establish whether you should supplement your diet.

FAT is our last macronutrient, and even though it has a bad reputation, you need fat for many important bodily functions. Now wait! This is not me telling you to eat an entire stick of butter.

Even though you need a certain amount of fat in your diet to help absorb certain vitamins, provide insulation for vital organs, and deliver essential fatty acids, just like the other macronutrients, some sources are more nutritious than others. Unlike the other macronutrients, you rarely have to make a concerted effort to include fat on your plate because it's found in many foods you're already eating, especially animal products.

We often talk about fats in terms of "good fat" and "bad fat." Bad fat refers to saturated fat, which our body needs in small amounts, but in excess can cause cardiovascular harm. Good fat refers to unsaturated fat, which actually improves cardiovascular health, promotes good brain function, and fights inflammation. An easy way to remember saturated vs. unsaturated fat is that saturated fat is solid at room temperature (like butter) while unsaturated fat is liquid at room temperature (like olive oil).

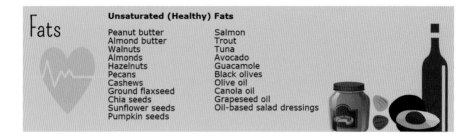

Fats

Unsaturated (Healthy) Fats

Peanut butter	Salmon
Almond butter	Trout
Walnuts	Tuna
Almonds	Avocado
Hazelnuts	Guacamole
Pecans	Black olives
Cashews	Olive oil
Ground flaxseed	Canola oil
Chia seeds	Grapeseed oil
Sunflower seeds	Oil-based salad dressings
Pumpkin seeds	

It's advisable to limit the amount of saturated fats you get in your diet. Sources of saturated fats include: whole milk, cream, butter, cheese, processed meats such as bacon, salami, and pepperoni, higher-fat cuts of beef and pork, and the skin on chicken or turkey.

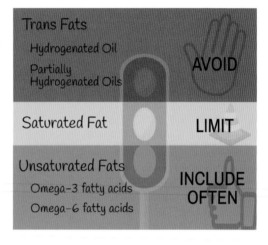

Trans Fats
Hydrogenated Oil
Partially Hydrogenated Oils — AVOID

Saturated Fat — LIMIT

Unsaturated Fats
Omega-3 fatty acids
Omega-6 fatty acids — INCLUDE OFTEN

On the other hand, you do want to include unsaturated fat in your diet daily—but remember, the calories add up quickly, so eat these foods in moderation! Check out the chart below for some of the best sources of unsaturated, or healthy, fats.

While you're limiting saturated fat, it's worth mentioning that there is one kind of fat that is especially bad for you called trans fat, which comes from hydrogenated and partially hydrogenated oils. While you may not be able to avoid these completely, it's a good practice to avoid them as much as possible, and really only include them in the occasional "fun food."

Examples of foods high in hydrogenated oils and trans fats include fried foods, frozen pizzas, biscuits, cakes and cookies, some crackers, and stick margarine.

Be cautious when evaluating products for trans fats. The Nutrition Facts label may say the product has 0 grams of trans fats, but that's per serving. It's not uncommon for companies to "hide" them. How's that? They only have to put it on the label if it's more than half a gram/serving, so if one serving of crackers has 0.45 grams of trans fat and you eat two servings, you've just eaten almost 1 gram of trans fat while you thought you were eating 0! It may not seem like a lot, but trans fats can be so detrimental to your health, the American Heart Association recommends eating 2 grams or less of trans fats per day. You can find these sneaky fats by looking for hydrogenated or partially hydrogenated oils on the ingredients list. Common offenders are crackers, chips, and flour tortillas.

Trend alert! Coconut oil is super popular and gaining lots of momentum on the "healthy fats" front . . . after all, it comes from a fruit, right? Yet it is solid at room temperature, which means it's a saturated fat. Confused? Me too. Coconut oil is very much a saturated fat, but because of the length of its triglycerides, preliminary research has shown its potential to have positive health effects. I won't bore you with the scientific details, but the bottom line is: More research is needed before

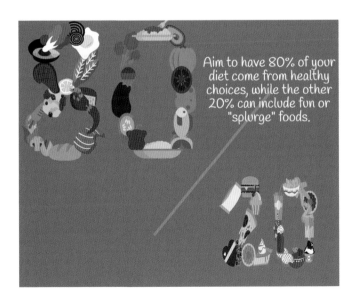

Aim to have 80% of your diet come from healthy choices, while the other 20% can include fun or "splurge" foods.

we go putting it into everything, and like any fat it should be used in moderation.

No, you don't have to give up _____.
The good news is that a well-balanced diet won't just have an appropriate mix of carbohydrate, protein, and fat. It will also have a nice balance of healthy foods and "fun" foods.

I often use the 80/20 rule, which simply means that 80 percent of the time we should be choosing healthy, nutrient-rich foods. The other twenty percent can be those fun foods that we enjoy and that we crave—bacon, donuts, burger and fries, pepperoni pizza, milkshakes—because including fun foods keep us from going totally crazy.

But choose your condiments wisely.
The healthiest choices to spice up your hot dogs, burgers, or fries are things like mustard or hot sauce, but that doesn't mean you have to throw out your ketchup and mayo. Just know that there are more healthy and less healthy versions out there.

Ketchup has had a bad reputation ever since news dropped that the leading brands are loaded with corn syrup and/or high-fructose corn syrup. Thankfully, companies have responded by offering healthier versions (Simply Heinz, Annie's Organic Ketchup, Hunt's 100% Natural, to name a few), but they're still relatively high in cane sugar, so you'll still want to use ketchup in moderation.

Mayonnaise is a bit trickier. Natural homemade mayo (made of eggs, seed/vegetable oil, vinegar, mustard) is actually quite healthy (again in moderation, as it's high in fat), but let's be serious, most of us are not going to whip up a batch of our own. Healthier store-bought versions do exist (such as Primal Kitchen's Avocado Oil Mayo, Sir Kensington's Organic Mayo, or the popular vegan option Just Mayo) but won't have the Hellman's or Miracle Whip taste you're probably craving. If that's you, go ahead and indulge, but either limit the amount you use or how often you're using it. Remember, eat the foods you love—balance is key.

5

WHAT'S ON YOUR PLATE?

So how does all this translate into what your plate should look like at each meal? We've been talking about carbohydrate, protein, and fat, but I'm going to switch it up slightly now. Don't panic. This will make it easier, I promise.

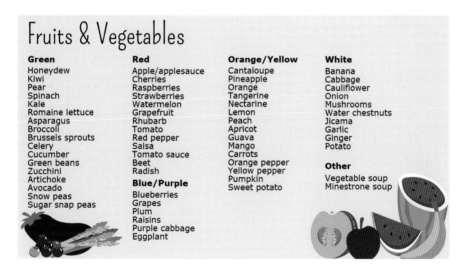

Fruits & Vegetables

Green	Red	Orange/Yellow	White
Honeydew	Apple/applesauce	Cantaloupe	Banana
Kiwi	Cherries	Pineapple	Cabbage
Pear	Raspberries	Orange	Cauliflower
Spinach	Strawberries	Tangerine	Onion
Kale	Watermelon	Nectarine	Mushrooms
Romaine lettuce	Grapefruit	Lemon	Water chestnuts
Asparagus	Rhubarb	Peach	Jicama
Broccoli	Tomato	Apricot	Garlic
Brussels sprouts	Red pepper	Guava	Ginger
Celery	Salsa	Mango	Potato
Cucumber	Tomato sauce	Carrots	
Green beans	Beet	Orange pepper	**Other**
Zucchini	Radish	Yellow pepper	
Artichoke		Pumpkin	Vegetable soup
Avocado	**Blue/Purple**	Sweet potato	Minestrone soup
Snow peas	Blueberries		
Sugar snap peas	Grapes		
	Plum		
	Raisins		
	Purple cabbage		
	Eggplant		

When it comes to your plate, we're going to change our categories to: carbohydrate, protein, and fruits and vegetables. Even though fruits and *some* vegetables are carb-rich, they get their own category on our plate because they are SO important. Not only are they packed with vitamins and minerals, they're also an important source of fiber. Best of all, they're generally low-calorie so we can load up on them without throwing off our energy balance—that's when your calorie intake is equal to the calories that you burn, which keeps body weight stable.

Adults need 2 cups of fruit and 2½ cups of vegetables each day for good health. Most Americans do not meet this recommendation.

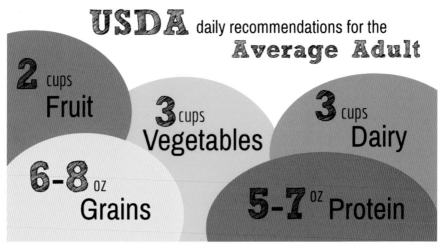

Ranges indicate the different needs for men and women, with men at the higher end of the range.
Source: United States Department of Agriculture 2015-2020 Dietary Guidelines for Americans
https://health.gov/dietaryguidelines/2015/guidelines/
https://www.choosemyplate.gov/MyPlate

VARIETY = THE SPICE OF LIFE

We've talked about balance, but aiming for *variety* within each food group will help to ensure that you're getting a wide range of nutrients—and make your mealtimes more interesting, as a bonus. It can be easy to gravitate toward the same foods week in and week out, especially if you have a busy schedule or if you're just learning your way around the kitchen. Challenge yourself to make an effort to vary the foods that you eat. Here are some ideas to help you break out of some common food ruts:

Carb-rich foods: Don't just rely on pasta and brown rice. Include starchy vegetables, quinoa, or wild rice. If you have a sandwich for lunch, don't always grab the same whole-wheat bread. Try it on a whole-wheat tortilla or pita bread.

Protein-rich foods: I often see athletes who eat chicken, chicken, and more chicken. Your protein-rich choices should absolutely include lean choices like chicken and turkey, but lots of other proteins offer additional benefits. Include fish and seafood to get healthy omega-3 fatty acids. Include beef and pork to increase iron intake. Include non-meat sources to cut down on total cholesterol intake and for additional fiber and antioxidants. A balanced diet will have a combination of many different proteins.

Fruits and Vegetables: These tend to have similar vitamin and mineral content based on their color. So, even though an orange pepper and a carrot are very different, they are both high in vitamins A and C because they are similarly colored. This means it's a good practice to include every color—red, orange, yellow, purple, blue, green, white—over the course of a week. If you regularly include lots of color and variety, you will likely be getting all the vitamins and minerals you need. If you do this consistently, you probably don't need to even bother with a multivitamin.

Athlete case files

When Amy, one of my student athletes, walked me through her normal diet, she admitted that most nights of the week for dinner she would eat a cold can of tuna, rice, and canned green beans. Wait . . . what?! Why? In probing further, I learned that her rather strange dinner choices were due to her lack of confidence in the kitchen: those were simply the easiest things for her to make.

In itself, her meal choice is a healthy one, however eating it nearly every day presented a couple of problems: First, her diet lacked variety, which means she was getting a limited subset of each macronutrient and thus a limited selection of vitamins and minerals. Second, tuna, although a nice protein choice in moderation, does contain small amounts of mercury, which can actually cause health problems if consumed in excess.

Amy and I talked about other quick (and cheap) proteins that she could add into her diet to replace her trusty can of tuna. Canned chicken, eggs, and even plant sources like beans and legumes were easy, low-cost items that she could have on hand. Additionally, we found one night each week that she could cook for the rest of the week, which would allow her to quickly add chicken breasts or ground beef or turkey to things like tacos or pasta sauce. Lastly, Amy agreed she could try to include a fresh veggie once or twice a week, expand her canned options past just green beans, and keep some frozen options on hand as well.

Normal Human Meal

Exactly what your plate should look like will vary a little based on your lifestyle, but to meet the nutritional needs for most Normal Humans (remember, that's you now) your plate should look similar to this:

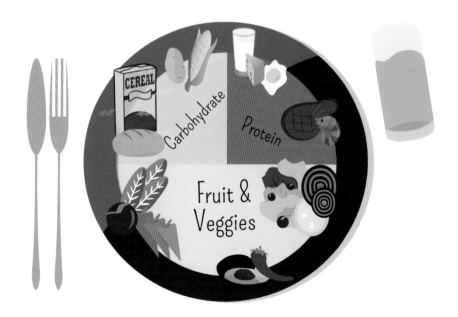

Filling half of your plate with fruits and vegetables ensures that you'll get plenty of fiber and a nice variety of vitamins and minerals. Plus, you can eat a lot of them without throwing off energy balance.

The quarter of your plate dedicated to carbohydrates should be where you include a grain like pasta or rice or starchy vegetable like potatoes or corn.

Lastly, the quarter of your plate dedicated to protein is where you can include meat, dairy, eggs, or plant-based proteins like beans.

Using this approach will ensure that you have all the macronutrients accounted for on your plate, but helps keep portion size in check.

For Those Heavy Lifters

If you still do heavy resistance training or train similarly to how you did as an athlete, that may warrant a slight increase to your carbohydrate and protein consumption.

Adequate protein will help support the muscle building that your training is designed to promote. Carbohydrates will help to ensure that you're intaking enough calories to support that muscle growth as well as replace energy stores.

This can be achieved simply by slightly increasing portion sizes of whichever protein and carbohydrate-rich food you choose for your meal. If bigger portions don't appeal to you, you could instead add a side that is rich in both protein and carbohydrate—a glass of milk, a cup of yogurt, a side of beans, or a protein bar if you're on the go. Meanwhile, always ensure that the last third of your plate is dedicated to a variety of fruits and vegetables.

If you have included regular heavy workouts in your plan, your plate should look more like this:

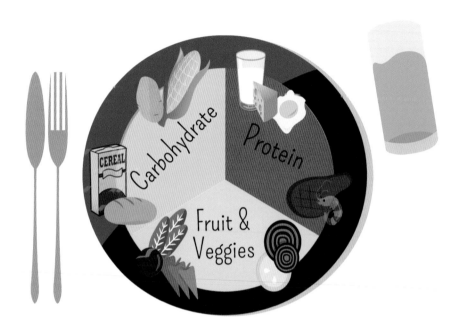

For The Super-Trainers

If you are completely out of your mind and still have joints that can take the abuse of doing something like a marathon, triathlon, ultra-trail, or Ironman, you probably need to increase your carbohydrate consumption to ensure your body has the appropriate amount of fuel. You'll want to aim for this increased carbohydrate intake during times of heavy training and competition.

(You may also want to go ahead and pencil in an appointment with an orthopedic surgeon, just in case you need new joints sooner than the rest of us.)

Note that this plate is not appropriate for leisurely runners (or swimmers or cyclists), even if you go for the occasional long run (swim, cycle).

This plate is reserved for those who are consistently running (swimming, cycling . . .) very high mileage and doing heavy and consistent training.

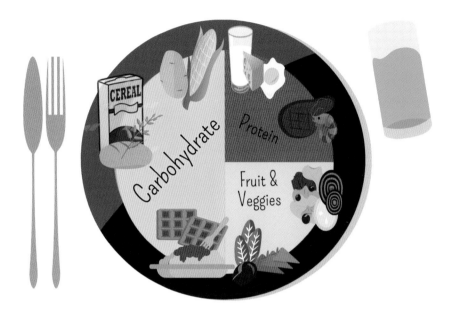

6

WHEN TO EAT

We've talked about what to eat and how much to eat, but what about when to eat it?

This is actually a very important piece of the nutrition puzzle—for both athletes and Normal Humans. In fact, for the athletes I work with, one of the simplest changes I urge them to make is to eat frequently and to never skip meals. It sometimes takes a little planning to make it happen, but timing can make a huge difference.

So why is something so simple so important? In the sports nutrition world, we often use the term "fuel" when it comes to food, because it truly is fueling our bodies.

With the same principle in mind, you can think of your body like a car that needs that fuel (food) to keep going. There is one inherent difference however: When your car runs out of gas, it stops.

Luckily, your body doesn't just stop moving and working if you haven't given it fuel in a while. What your body DOES do is break down fuel that you've stored so it can continue to function. Now, if your body only used stored fat for this purpose, that would be ideal, but it doesn't. It breaks down stored carbohydrate and also protein (aka muscle).

Remember we talked about how you should hold on to as much muscle as you can since it's a little harder to come by these days?

So here's my advice: Eat frequently.

You should be eating a small meal or snack every 3 to 4 hours. This will help for a number of reasons:

1. It will help you stay full.
2. It will help prevent cravings and overeating.
3. It will help you maintain optimal body composition by preserving muscle and stimulating fat burn.
4. It will help promote a faster metabolism.

Don't forget though, the "what" and the "how much" are still important. If you eat a McDonald's cheeseburger and fries every 4 hours then you probably aren't going to meet your goals.

And, as always, at each of these frequent meals and snacks, it's important to maintain balance between carbohydrate and protein, include fruits and veggies, and watch portion sizes.

Also keep in mind that, unless you are keeping up heavy endurance training, your body is undergoing some pretty big changes. You might think that it would be happy to slow down a bit and cruise—after all, how many times did you find yourself actually apologizing out loud to your body for everything your sport was putting it through?—but sometimes it takes a while before your body catches up to those changes and makes the necessary adjustments, as you'll see in the next case file:

Athlete case files

Monica had recently finished her final season of competitive swimming and was working to adjust her diet for her new Normal Human lifestyle. She had developed sound nutrition habits for a college athlete, but 4 to 5 hours of training in the pool each day meant she still had to eat *a lot*. Monica was concerned because she felt she had appropriately reduced her food intake for her decreased activity level, but she often felt like she was starving. It seemed her appetite hadn't caught up with the lifestyle change.

These kinds of exercise and appetite imbalances are actually pretty common when activity levels change drastically. In fact, some retired athletes experience the exact opposite—their appetite decreases so much due to the lower activity that they have trouble eating enough because they're simply not hungry. The good news is that these mismatches tend to work themselves out eventually if you stay the course.

In Monica's case, we agreed first that she should still aim to eat every 3–4 hours and that she should really try to stick to that "schedule" to help her body (and metabolism) get into a routine. Second, she shouldn't ignore her hunger cues completely. While it's likely that her hunger was misled to some extent, hunger is your body's way of telling you what it needs. I advised her to stick to her current portions, but if 20–30 minutes passed after a meal and she was still hungry to consider having a little more of the balanced meal she had planned or a healthy snack.

Don't be surprised if you find yourself in a similar situation for the first few months after retirement. If you feel like your hunger is much more extreme than it should be given your activity level, make sure you're adequately hydrating and including plenty of fiber and protein in your diet—both of which can help keep you full longer. If the hunger feels tied to boredom or emotional eating, try to distract yourself by going on a walk, calling a friend or family member, or doing something else that you enjoy. If the hunger, or lack of hunger, ever feels out of control or you notice that you've gained or lost a large amount of weight (more than 1 to 2 pounds per week for multiple weeks), seek out the help of a dietitian or physician.

As mentioned in the case file with Monica, how much to eat and when to eat it doesn't always feel natural right off the bat. However, once you settle into your Normal Human routine and develop good habits with healthy eating and exercise patterns, my hope is that you start to listen to your body and move toward what we in the biz call "intuitive eating." Simply put, intuitive eating focuses on listening to your body when it comes to things like hunger cues and fullness levels, and encourages focusing on your health and happiness instead of just weight. A couple fellow dietitians wrote an excellent book on this exact topic called *Intuitive Eating*. It would make an excellent Normal Human purchase if you feel like this is right up your alley.

7

HYDRATION

This is a term you should be used to, and I'm not referring to the "hydration" practiced on weekends at Kappa Delta Sig. It was likely preached by your coaching staff, your training staff, and your dietitian if you had one. Hydration is still important as a Normal Human, but it'll look a little different now.

Hydration for an elite athlete is often a game of keeping up. You can surely recall bringing your water bottle wherever you went (to have a chance of replacing the fluid you lost as a sweaty mess at practice), but wondering if it was worth it as you headed for the Ladies or Gents room for the 15th time that day.

As a Normal Human, proper hydration still does you a lot of good by helping you to:

✓ Optimize your metabolism
✓ Keep your GI tract healthy
✓ Be more aware of hunger and fullness cues

The popular "eight 8-ounce glasses per day" guideline is a good starting point for most individuals. If you tend to sweat quite a bit during your workouts, it will likely be more.

Drinking 64 ounces of fluid each day may seem easy-peasy, but remember, there are no more Athletic Training students standing by to hand you a water bottle at a moment's notice.

Here are a few tips for making sure you get enough fluids in each day:

1. Drink a glass of water first thing in the morning. This is a common time to neglect, because even if you wake up with your mouth feeling like the Sahara Desert, you may brush your teeth or eat breakfast and then forget about it.

2. Keep a refillable water bottle at your desk (or wherever your job allows).

3. Take bottled water with you when you go to work or out to run errands so you're less likely to stop and get a not-so-healthy beverage. You might even want to try buying a 64-ounce bottle, filling it in the morning, and keeping it with you throughout the day so you can track whether or not you're meeting your daily fluid intake needs.

4. If you're not a huge fan of water and crave a "taste" in your beverages, try adding lemon, lime, cucumber, or unsweetened frozen fruit to your water.

5. Download a free app such as Waterlogged, My Water Balance, Plant Nanny, or Drink Water Reminder—to name a few—to nag you into it.

6. If you feel hungry shortly after eating a meal or a snack, ensure that you're adequately hydrated. Sometimes thirst is misconceived as hunger!

BALANCE YOUR BEVERAGES

Some drinks are far better choices than others. If you're not careful, beverages are a very easy way to rack up calories (see page 55) without really filling you up like food would, and often with no nutritional value.

Besides empty calories, certain beverages have other negative side effects. Sugary beverages like soda, lemonade, sweet tea, and even sports drinks like Gatorade and Powerade can harm your teeth and promote tooth decay. Carbonated beverages, even naturally fizzy water such as San Pellegrino, get those bubbles from carbonic acid, which breaks down tooth enamel over time. Add the sugar in sodas into that equation and the damage to your teeth multiplies. Additionally, consumption of soda (including diet soda!) has been linked to lower bone density, especially in women.

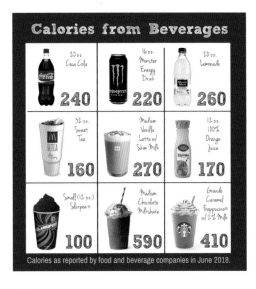

The occasional soda or carbonated water won't make your teeth fall out or set you on a straight path to osteoporosis, but if you drink these regularly and/or in large quantities, you may want to start weaning yourself off them for healthier options.

One beverage to limit that deserves its very own paragraph is energy drinks. Not only are these carbonated sugar bombs, they're loaded with caffeine—which teams up with the sugar to give you an unsustainable burst of energy, usually followed by an energy slump or crash. Energy drinks are also poorly regulated by the FDA because they are considered supplements rather than food. If Red Bull or 5-Hour Energy is the only thing keeping you awake at the wheel, the occasional energy drink is better than crashing into a tree, but these should definitely be limited in your diet as much as possible.

Athlete case files

Brittany was working on losing a few pounds, but struggling. I had her keep a food log for 3 days, tracking everything she ate and all of her workouts. After analyzing her data, I was puzzled. Based on her workouts, she *should* have been losing some weight if she was consistently following the diet she wrote down, which she insisted she was doing, so I probed a little further. "I noticed you didn't write down any beverages—does that mean you were only drinking water?" I asked. "Well . . . no . . ." she replied slowly.

We went through her diet again, this time adding in the beverages. Every morning she had a Grande Caramel Macchiato from Starbucks, at lunch usually a lemonade or fruit juice, and dinner most nights included her favorite, sweet tea. Brittany thought she was approaching her beverages in a healthy manner. After all, it's not like she was drinking soda every day. We discussed how quickly these calories add up, even in seemingly innocent drinks: 250 calories in her macchiato, another 300 in her fruit juice, and nearly 250 in her sweet tea. She was consuming 800 calories a day just from drinks— certainly enough to keep her from meeting her weight loss goals!

Water wasn't a favorite for Brittany, so we discussed some other options: Infusing water with fruit, cucumber, or mint, switching to unsweetened tea (or at least slowly weaning herself off the heavily sweetened kind), drinking coffee instead of blended coffee drinks, and trying various flavored water products. Once Brittany changed her beverage habits, her weight loss goals became much more attainable and those few pounds actually came off pretty quickly.

Alcohol (this is an important one!)

When it comes to racking up calories from beverages, the easiest place to do so is at the bar. Since you have presumably just completed or are about to complete your collegiate or professional sports career, I'm operating under the assumption that by now you know that alcohol has the ability to be delicious and fun—as well as nausea-provoking and spiteful.

Here's the problem with our friend alcohol: By its very nature, it is high in calories. As in, the molecule that makes you drunk has 7 calories/gram (almost as much as fat has at 9 calories/gram). Now add in sugar-heavy mixers like juice, soda, syrup, or fat-heavy cream. That's right, your favorite cocktail is almost certainly extremely high in calories.

Alcohol doesn't just rack up calories, though. It's a powerful diuretic, which, quite simply, makes you pee. *(Think back to all those long restroom lines at the bar . . .)* That also means it causes dehydration and that dehydration is what gives you a killer headache the next morning. *(Heads up: Hangovers will be worse the older you get, promise.)*

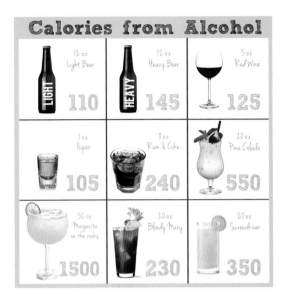

We haven't even gotten to the worst part yet.

Once you've gotten good and liquored up, made questionable decisions *(a whole other topic for someone else's book)*, and effectively dehydrated yourself, you *will* be hungry. That's because alcohol also stimulates hunger, and you probably won't stop off for a 3 a.m. salad or healthy smoothie. Calories from "drunk food" contribute significantly to the overall surplus for the night—a surplus that can easily be 2,000-3,000 calories more than you need for the day.

Now, before you go to angrily pour yourself a tall one to forget about the mean dietitian saying how bad drinking can be, I'm not saying that you should never drink alcohol. After all, we've already identified that it can be delicious and fun.

Rather, just like food, I suggest you approach alcohol in moderation and use a few tips to help negate calories where possible:

1. **Remember that moderation = 1 drink/day for women and 2 drinks/day for men.** *(Note: these do not function like rollover minutes on your cell phone.)* One drink = one 12-ounce beer or one 5-ounce glass of wine or one 1.5-ounce shot of liquor. Your body metabolizes

alcohol at a rate of about 1 drink/hour. This rate can vary slightly with gender, age, and size, but not by as much as you'd think.

2. **Avoid high-calorie mixers like soda, tonic, juice, syrups, pre-made drink mixes, energy drinks, and cream.** Instead, mix with water, lemon or lime juice, soda water, or diet soda.

3. **If you plan to drink a lot, include some nonalcoholic drinks throughout the night.** Water is an excellent choice. This will also help to reduce the magnitude of your hangover.

4. **Have a plan for drunk food.** Identify the healthiest late-night food options near your favorite bars and/or have pre-portioned healthy leftovers, a small microwave meal, or individual thin pizza ready at home to satisfy cravings without going totally overboard on calories.

5. **Focus on enjoying the company you're with, rather than focusing on drinking.**

6. **Set limits for yourself such as only drinking alcohol on weekends.** If you have friends in town or a special event to celebrate mid-week, you can always make an exception to the rule, but by abstaining during the workweek most of the time, you'll maximize your productivity and minimize your calorie consumption.

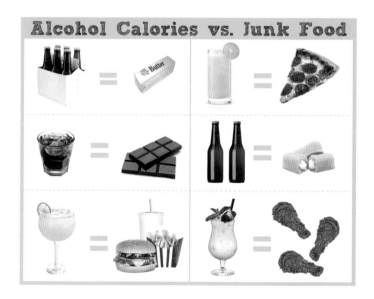

Practicing some of these tips will not only help you to be a more functional Normal Human, it can also help you save some money. Drinks at restaurants and bars are usually expensive, which means they add up quickly in the calorie *and* cost departments!

And in case you still need convincing, the graphic on page 58 provides some sobering math on how quickly calories from alcohol add up. Note: while I use these calorie comparisons to make a point, remember that I'm not implying you should never eat these foods. Everyone needs some pizza in their life—I feel strongly about that.

SO . . . WHAT *SHOULD* YOU BE DRINKING?

The beverage you should be choosing most often is *water*. This should come as no surprise—it's pure, hydrating, and calorie-free. While water is great, it doesn't mean it's the only healthy beverage out there, nor does it mean that it's the only fluid that helps hydrate you.

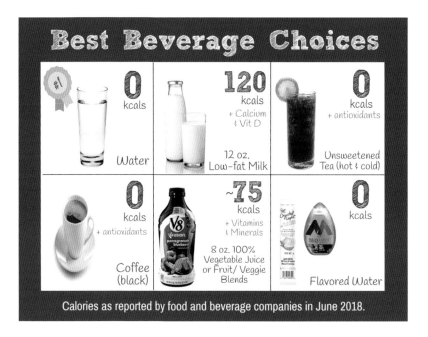

Your other options do come with caveats though.

Black coffee and *unsweetened tea* (hot or cold) are nice calorie-free options, and they come with the added benefit of antioxidants, which help manage inflammation. Notice that I said *black* coffee and *unsweetened* tea—if you go and dump a bunch of sugar and/or cream into either one, the calories start to add up quickly.

Additionally, unless the label states otherwise, most varieties of coffee and tea (even green tea) contain caffeine. Caffeine is great to help perk you up for that early Monday meeting, but everyone metabolizes it differently, so don't abuse amounts of these beverages. For most people, 8 to 16 ounces/day is reasonable, but pay attention to how caffeine affects you. If you're getting headaches, chest pains, or stomach pain, discontinue your caffeine use until you talk to a doctor.

Other beverages that can be included regularly as part of a healthy diet are *low-fat milk* (skim, 1%, or 2%) and *100 percent vegetable juice or fruit and veggie juice blends. (Note: Hi-C and fruit punch packets are* not *100 percent juice.)* These options contain a fair amount of calories, so keep that in mind, but they both offer additional health benefits as well. Milk provides protein, calcium, and vitamin D and can help you feel fuller, while fruit and veggie juices provide vitamins and antioxidants.

Flavored water is also a great option to "spice up" your hydration routine. Flavoring water naturally with fruit, mint, or cucumber is ideal, but store-bought packets can be handy as well. These tend to contain artificial sweeteners however, so use these in moderation.

As with every aspect of your diet, practicing moderation and variety are key when it comes to your Normal Human hydration plan. Are you sensing a theme yet? Yes, balance, that's right!

Oh and if you want to be my favorite, I also suggest buying a reusable water bottle and coffee thermos. The paper and plastic consumption from beverages is pretty out of control in many parts of the world, and every little bit helps . . .

8

SMART GROCERY SHOPPING

Hopefully at this point in your life you have at least some experience with grocery shopping. Unfortunately if you're like most college students, it was probably sporadic and involved grocery carts filled with whatever looked and sounded good in the moment—usually not very healthy items.

As a Normal Human, you should plan to go to the grocery store at least once every week or two. The more often you go, the more fresh fruits and veggies you can buy, and the less likely you will be to rely on processed or frozen foods. It can also help avoid wasting food—and wasted food is wasted money (and not nice for the environment).

The first and most important step of grocery shopping happens way before you even set foot in the store—making a list!

Believe it or not, the simple step of making a list is the most basic form of meal planning. Taking the time to put together a grocery list will help ensure that you leave with everything you need, and that you don't buy a bunch of stuff you really could have done without.

It may be helpful to keep a running list on the fridge or counter or on your phone so that you can jot down items you run out of during the week. When it's time to make your grocery list, you'll already have a couple of items that you know you'll need to grab.

From there, ask yourself, "What will I eat for breakfast this week?" You know you need a carbohydrate, protein, and some fruit or veggies if possible (go back to the charts in chapter 4 if you need help deciding which carbs and proteins would make good breakfast options for you). Write these down. Repeat this process for lunch and dinner and write down a couple of healthy snack options as well.

When I bring up the topic of "meal planning" with my athletes, it's usually met with wide-eyed stares. I imagine that's because they are picturing a scenario in which they'll be required to have 47 carefully labeled plastic containers sprawled out across the table and kitchen counter with premeasured amounts of each food.

Don't panic. What I'm suggesting is a far cry from that.

Breakfast and lunch tend to be easier because we can generally eat the same one or two things for these meals over the course of a week. Dinner is usually the intimidating meal when it comes to planning. My suggestion is to start by choosing two meals you can make for dinner that week.

If you're not an experienced cook, start simple—choose things like tacos, spaghetti, or chicken and rice. Whichever two things you choose, I suggest making more than you'll eat in one sitting. By doubling or tripling batches, it not only gives you leftovers for another dinner that week, but you can also use those leftovers for quick lunches, which we'll talk about more in the next chapter. Leftovers may not be glamorous, but eating them will save you money and lighten your cooking load considerably.

You may even want to plan to make more of just the protein rather than the entire meal. By cooking a bunch of chicken at one time for instance—on the grill, in the oven, or even in a slow cooker (see recipe on page 103)—you can speed up meal prep later in the week. You can throw the chicken in a stir-fry or pasta for a quick dinner or use it to make a sandwich or wrap for lunch. A little planning ahead opens up all kinds of possibilities. This is a great practice to get into, especially if you've got a busy schedule or just tend to be lazy in the kitchen.

With a well-thought-out grocery list in hand, it's time to head to the store!

Here are some tips to get the most out of your trip:

1. **Start with the perimeter of the store**

   This is where most of the fresh food is found—fruits and vegetables, deli, fresh meat and seafood, dairy, and the bakery (skip the cakes and focus on whole-grain breads).

2. **Be smart when buying fruits and vegetables**

   ✓ Buy produce that's in season. For example, berries are in season during the summer—which means during those months they'll taste great and cost less. In the winter, berries will be much more expensive and probably not nearly as tasty. Besides cost and quality, a good indicator of what's in season in your region is where the produce was grown—if it's local, it's likely in season.

   ✓ Buy only what you will use in a 1- to 2-week span to avoid throwing out a bunch of stuff that went bad.

   ✓ Vary the kinds of produce you're buying. Some produce goes bad quickly, while some can last quite some time in the pantry or fridge. Aim to buy a combination, and eat the produce that won't last as long first.

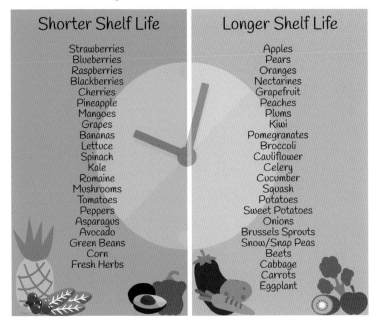

Shorter Shelf Life	Longer Shelf Life
Strawberries	Apples
Blueberries	Pears
Raspberries	Oranges
Blackberries	Nectarines
Cherries	Grapefruit
Pineapple	Peaches
Mangoes	Plums
Grapes	Kiwi
Bananas	Pomegranates
Lettuce	Broccoli
Spinach	Cauliflower
Kale	Celery
Romaine	Cucumber
Mushrooms	Squash
Tomatoes	Potatoes
Peppers	Sweet Potatoes
Asparagus	Onions
Avocado	Brussels Sprouts
Green Beans	Snow/Snap Peas
Corn	Beets
Fresh Herbs	Cabbage
	Carrots
	Eggplant

✓ Store fruits and vegetables appropriately. This will help them stay fresh as long as possible. For instance, did you know:

- That tomatoes should be kept on the counter, and not in the fridge?
- That potatoes and onions should be kept in a cool, dark place like a pantry?
- That some fruits, such as apples and bananas, produce a gas called ethylene that makes other produce ripen more quickly? Which is great if you're trying to get that peach to ripen more quickly, but not ideal if you're wondering why your fruit bowl doesn't seem to last long before things start getting fuzzy.

Check out this guide to how to best store your fresh produce:

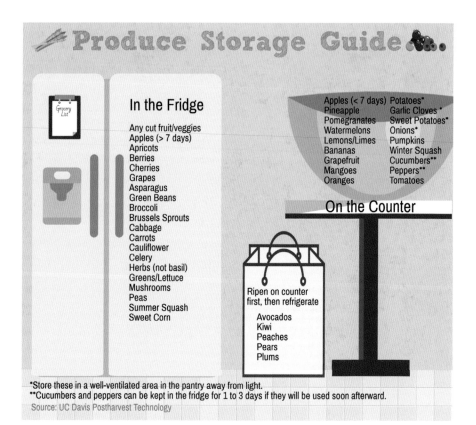

Produce Storage Guide

In the Fridge

Any cut fruit/veggies
Apples (> 7 days)
Apricots
Berries
Cherries
Grapes
Asparagus
Green Beans
Broccoli
Brussels Sprouts
Cabbage
Carrots
Cauliflower
Celery
Herbs (not basil)
Greens/Lettuce
Mushrooms
Peas
Summer Squash
Sweet Corn

Apples (< 7 days)	Potatoes*
Pineapple	Garlic Cloves *
Pomegranates	Sweet Potatoes*
Watermelons	Onions*
Lemons/Limes	Pumpkins
Bananas	Winter Squash
Grapefruit	Cucumbers**
Mangoes	Peppers**
Oranges	Tomatoes

On the Counter

Ripen on counter first, then refrigerate

Avocados
Kiwi
Peaches
Pears
Plums

*Store these in a well-ventilated area in the pantry away from light.
**Cucumbers and peppers can be kept in the fridge for 1 to 3 days if they will be used soon afterward.
Source: UC Davis Postharvest Technology

✓ Weigh the costs and benefits of buying precut/prewashed produce. It will almost always be more expensive and won't stay fresh as long, so generally unwashed whole fruits and veggies are your best bet. However, be realistic with your schedule and abilities. If you have a crazy week ahead and know you won't have time to prep certain produce, it may be worth the higher cost to buy the pre-prepped ones. Maybe you love pomegranates, but don't have the first clue how to cut/shuck one. Buy the pre-shucked pomegranate until you have time to YouTube how to do it yourself. At the end of the day, you want to make sure you're getting enough fruits and vegetables in your diet—so figure out the most realistic way to make that happen.

3. **Buy protein items on sale**

Proteins are usually the most expensive items in your grocery cart, so if you can find them on sale, take advantage! Consider buying more than you normally would and putting some in the freezer. Also be open to trying cheaper cuts of meat. For beef and pork, that may mean that they're not as lean, but depending on what you're using it for you may be able to trim off some of that fat. We all love filet mignon, but a flank steak will be more affordable and probably still delicious. Chicken is a great example as well— chicken breasts are great, lean protein options, but they're substantially pricier than legs and thighs. If you remove the skin from the legs and thighs, they're still tasty lean protein sources, and they will cost half as much (or less) than breasts. You can also cut very large chicken breasts in half or sometimes even thirds to keep portion sizes and cost in check.

4. **Buy items in bulk to save**

But don't go too crazy with this suggestion. Especially if you're only feeding a family of one, buying in bulk might not make sense. It is usually cheaper though, so if there are foods you eat often (cereal, pasta, or yogurt for example) and you're sure you'll eat it all before the expiration date, you'll get better value on the bigger sizes.

5. **Buy the store brand**

   The generic store brand will always be cheaper and for many items will be very similar to, if not the same as, the name brand.

6. **Skip the junk food aisles**

   Out of sight, out of mind. The best practice when it comes to avoiding junk food is to just not buy it! If this doesn't seem realistic compared to your current junk food consumption, try choosing just one "splurge" item when you go to the store. Maybe it's your favorite chips or a package of cookies you've been craving—whatever it is, also consider buying the smaller package. This can help control the amount being consumed.

7. **Consider buying frozen meat, fish, and produce**

   These can be nice alternatives if you run out of fresh options before your next trip to the store. Frozen fruits and veggies are cheaper and they are still great options nutritionally. They are especially nice in the winter when fresh produce might be more expensive or harder to find.

8. **Remember, not all premade meals are equal**

   If you feel you need to ease your way into the whole "cooking for yourself" thing or that you need no-hassle options on hand, there is a growing market for all-natural* premade frozen meals—that is, they're made from real, unprocessed food (often organic and sustainably sourced) with no artificial additives or preservatives. Look for brands such as Blake's, Kashi, Amy's Kitchen, Annie Chun's, or Trader Joe's. Even 100% chicken or fish nuggets can be a healthy protein choice.

9. **Join your grocery store's reward program**

   These are almost always free to join and can save you hundreds, if not thousands, of dollars over the course of a year.

Be aware that "natural" claims on food labels are not regulated. Make sure you check the ingredient list in the Nutrition Facts label (which is regulated).

Understanding Labels

Knowing how to read labels and being aware of sneaky marketing ploys are key to healthy eating. As consumers, we have a lot of decisions to make when we set foot in the grocery store. Companies know we're more concerned with knowing where our food comes from and making healthy choices than ever before, which means we're surrounded by a barrage of claims on packaging. Let's take a closer look at what it all means:

Label claims that *are* regulated by the FDA or USDA	
LOW-FAT	3 grams or less of fat in the given serving size.
FAT FREE	Less than 0.5 grams of total fat for a given serving size
LIGHT	50% reduction in fat for higher fat foods OR 33% reduction in calories for lower fat foods.
SUGAR FREE	Less than 0.5 grams of sugar for a given serving size
NO SUGAR ADDED	The manufacturer has not *added* any sugar to the product, however the product may have sugar naturally present.
SODIUM FREE	Less than 5 mg per labeled serving size
ORGANIC	Produce grown without the use of pesticides, synthetic fertilizers, sewage sludge, GMOs or ionizing radiation. Animals that produce meat, poultry, eggs, and dairy products do not take antibiotics or growth hormones.
HORMONE / ANTIBIOTIC FREE	Hormones and antibiotics were not used to speed the growth of the animal. Sometimes manufacturers use these products for short amounts of time, but discontinue use before they slaughter.
GLUTEN FREE	Does not contain gluten from barley, rye, or wheat in amounts exceeding 20 parts per million.

These labels do not necessarily mean the food in question is a *healthy* choice! Plenty of organic, GMO-free foods still have a high fat and added sugar content, such as organic double chocolate chip cookies. And low-fat or fat-free foods often have high levels of added sugar and/or sodium to make up for the flavor lost when they removed the fat.

Label claims that can be misleading	
FARM FRESH	Not regulated, completely meaningless.
CAGE FREE	This claim is regulated, so it does mean the chickens don't live in cages, but they can still be crowded into very tight quarters with thousands of other birds.
FREE RANGE OR FREE ROAMING	This claim is regulated, but the only requirement is that the animal is not caged and was allowed access to the outside. Often conditions mean the chickens never actually go outside. For natural eggs and poultry, look for an Organic, "Pasture Raised" label, which means the chickens actually spend most of their lives outside eating naturally. Unfortunately these will cost significantly more.
NATURAL OR ALL NATURAL	This claim is not currently regulated by the FDA, though it may be in the future. The USDA considers it to be a product containing no artificial ingredient or added color and only minimally processed (that is, processed in a manner that does not fundamentally alter the product) and labels must include a statement explaining why the term "natural" is used (such as "no artificial ingredients").
GMO FREE	This label is not regulated by the government and means nothing, however if a product has a "Non-GMO Project Verified" seal, it has been certified by the independent nonprofit organization as containing less than 0.9% GMO ingredients.

While packaging label claims such as those on the previous pages are not always regulated, the Nutrition Facts label is strictly regulated by the FDA—but there are still a few pitfalls to avoid. You're going to want to make sure you pay close attention to this label when you're shopping so you know what you're really putting on your plate.

Here are the different components of the label and what you should be looking for:

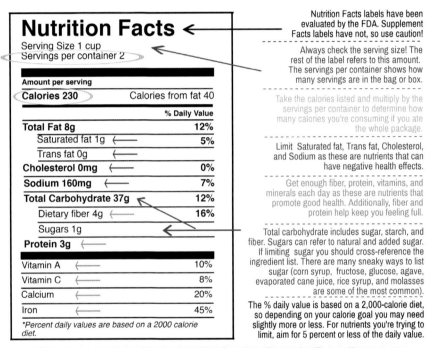

Nutrition Facts ←

Serving Size 1 cup
Servings per container 2

Amount per serving

Calories 230   Calories from fat 40

                                      % Daily Value

Total Fat 8g   **12%**

  Saturated fat 1g ←   **5%**

  Trans fat 0g ←

Cholesterol 0mg ←   **0%**

Sodium 160mg ←   **7%**

Total Carbohydrate 37g   **12%**

  Dietary fiber 4g ←   **16%**

  Sugars 1g

Protein 3g ←

Vitamin A ←   10%

Vitamin C ←   8%

Calcium ←   20%

Iron ←   45%

Percent daily values are based on a 2000 calorie diet.

Nutrition Facts labels have been evaluated by the FDA. Supplement Facts labels have not, so use caution!

Always check the serving size! The rest of the label refers to this amount. The servings per container shows how many servings are in the bag or box.

Take the calories listed and multiply by the servings per container to determine how many calories you're consuming if you ate the whole package.

Limit Saturated fat, Trans fat, Cholesterol, and Sodium as these are nutrients that can have negative health effects.

Get enough fiber, protein, vitamins, and minerals each day as these are nutrients that promote good health. Additionally, fiber and protein help keep you feeling full.

Total carbohydrate includes sugar, starch, and fiber. Sugars can refer to natural and added sugar. If limiting sugar you should cross-reference the ingredient list. There are many sneaky ways to list sugar (corn syrup, fructose, glucose, agave, evaporated cane juice, rice syrup, and molasses are some of the most common).

The % daily value is based on a 2,000-calorie diet, so depending on your calorie goal you may need slightly more or less. For nutrients you're trying to limit, aim for 5 percent or less of the daily value.

Ingredients: Be aware of foods with a long ingredient list or lots of long, scientific sounding names you don't recognize as food. These are both indications that the food may be highly processed. Also, be aware that ingredients are listed from most to least as they occur in the food. You want to see healthy ingredients listed first and things like sugar, high-fructose corn syrup, salt, and unhealthy fats listed toward the end.

Also remember to avoid foods that list hydrogenated or partially hydrogenated oils—those sources of dangerous trans fats—in the ingredients list.

Now that you have an idea of what to look for on a Nutrition Facts label, you should be aware that certain things about the label have recently undergone some pretty notable changes! Per the FDA, manufacturers had to make the switch by the summer of 2018. However, manufacturers with less than $10 million in annual sales will have an additional year to comply. The good news is that the changes are all in the consumer's best interest and are meant to help identify nutrients that are important to Americans' health.

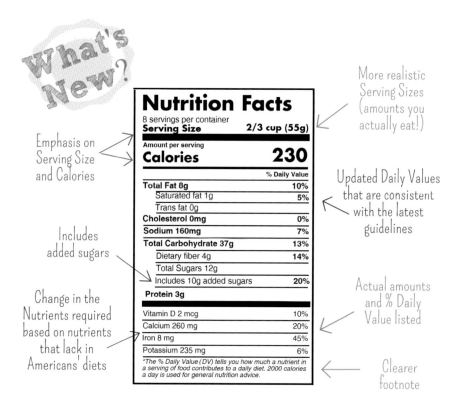

You can get more detailed information on the changes to the Nutrition Facts label on the FDA website via this link: goo.gl/iPPPfV.

9

PACKING A LUNCH

This throwback from your grade school days can be a gigantic money saver and a huge help nutritionally.

On average, Americans spend $7 to $12 every time they eat out for lunch. Even on the low end of that average, doing so every workday would cost you $35/week. That's $140/month or almost $1,700/year.

And from a nutrition standpoint, even a supposedly healthy lunch out like a salad or sandwich can add up quickly in the calorie column depending on the ingredients, which you don't typically have control over when you're eating out. What is that dressing or sauce made of? How much are they going to use?

With a little planning, you can save a good chunk of money and put yourself in a better spot nutritionally by packing your own lunch—and I promise it doesn't have to be complicated or take up much of your valuable adult time.

A good first step is to assess what equipment you'll have access to at work. Is there a fridge? A microwave? Will you need to bring your own knife, spoon, or fork?

These factors will all affect what kinds of food you should be packing (if there's no microwave, will you realistically eat cold or lukewarm leftovers or soup?) and what you should be packing it in.

Athlete case files

Most of my athletes could attest that I do indeed pack my lunch every single day, in my cute little Vera Bradley lunch bag. One day one of my athletes, Kenny, commented, "Why do you spend so much time bothering to pack a lunch when Subway and Jimmy John's are right across the street?"

While I do enjoy a good sub sandwich, I explained to Kenny that by packing my lunch I was consuming fewer calories but eating way more food. I also told him that I saved a ton of money by doing so. Kenny didn't believe me on either front, so I agreed that we would compare our lunches.

First we looked at calories. Every day for lunch, Kenny stopped at Subway and got a foot-long Sweet Onion Chicken Teriyaki sandwich (570 calories if he didn't add any other sauces or extras) and sometimes chips (250 calories) and a cookie (210 calories)—so over 1,000 calories just for lunch. This may be an acceptable number of lunch calories for Athlete Kenny, but it is probably too many calories for Normal Human Kenny.

Then I showed him what I had in my lunch bag: turkey and cheese on a whole-wheat tortilla (300 calories), Greek yogurt (100 calories), apple (70 calories), cucumbers and peppers (30 calories), and mandarin oranges (80 calories)—a total of 580 calories for generally more food, and more nutritious food at that!

Another big difference is how much we spent on our respective lunches. Kenny spent $10.11 for his foot-long sandwich, chips and a cookie. If he ate that every workday he would spend $50.55 in a week, $202.20 in a month, and $2,426.40 in a year. Whoa. That's a lot of money spent on lunch! (*Worth mentioning that number could be a little lower if he chose from the monthly $5 foot-long list.*)

On the other hand, my lunch cost me about $4—less than half of what Kenny was spending. After we broke it down, Kenny agreed that spending 5 to 10 minutes at night or in the morning to make his lunch at least a few days a week would be well worth it.

It will be helpful to invest in a lunch bag or lunchbox and individual-portion-size Tupperware or other reusable plastic containers. It might seem lame, but it will make your thoughtfully packed lunch much more enjoyable (crushed food is a bummer!) and help keep you from overeating by controlling portion size.

Have fun with it. Spoil yourself with that deluxe *Star Wars* lunch pail your parents wouldn't spring for or look into the growing market for cool and inventive lunch boxes for adults. If you're on a really tight budget, you can always wash and reuse sturdy containers from foods such as deli meats, yogurt, or cottage cheese instead of throwing them in the recycle bin.

Once you're ready to decide what to pack, remember that your goal is to aim for balance at each meal. You'll want to identify a protein, carbohydrate, and some fruit and/or vegetables to pack.

I recommend also packing a couple of healthy items that can be eaten as snacks in addition to your main lunch items. This is a great opportunity to ramp up fruit and veggie consumption. They're a great option for munching on during the day because the calories don't add up quickly, unlike most other munchies that you might gravitate toward.

Vegetables are also a great snack option for work because you are more or less stuck with what you've packed. This makes it much more likely that you'll eat them, whereas at home with all those choices it's much easier to talk yourself out of eating the veggies. Plus it provides a healthy alternative for those of you surrounded by vending machines or coworkers who are constantly bringing in donuts, cookies, and other high-cal nibbles.

If you don't enjoy veggies plain, try dipping them in hummus or a Greek yogurt-based dip. Just buy plain Greek yogurt and a packet of your favorite spices (such as French onion or the popular Hidden Valley Ranch) then mix for a much healthier version of the flavor you're craving. If you look at the ingredients list of most premade dips and salad dressings (the ones restaurants typically use as well!), you'll find that oils and sugar tend to top the list.

Packing your lunch is a great opportunity to be creative, but even if you're going to go back to basics and pack a sandwich, there are endless possibilities. Use whatever is on hand, especially the fresh meats and produce that are likely to spoil soonest and try new combinations to keep things interesting.

Here are some ideas and pointers on sandwich do's and don'ts:

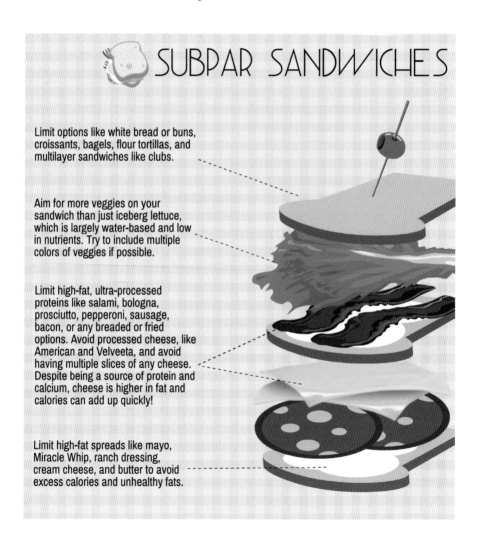

SUBPAR SANDWICHES

Limit options like white bread or buns, croissants, bagels, flour tortillas, and multilayer sandwiches like clubs.

Aim for more veggies on your sandwich than just iceberg lettuce, which is largely water-based and low in nutrients. Try to include multiple colors of veggies if possible.

Limit high-fat, ultra-processed proteins like salami, bologna, prosciutto, pepperoni, sausage, bacon, or any breaded or fried options. Avoid processed cheese, like American and Velveeta, and avoid having multiple slices of any cheese. Despite being a source of protein and calcium, cheese is higher in fat and calories can add up quickly!

Limit high-fat spreads like mayo, Miracle Whip, ranch dressing, cream cheese, and butter to avoid excess calories and unhealthy fats.

SUPERB SANDWICHES

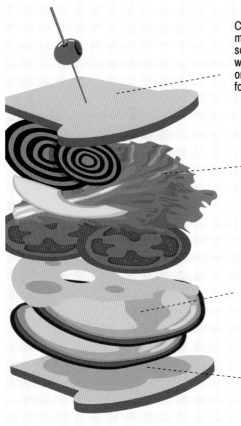

Choose options like whole-wheat or multigrain bread or buns, nut bread, sourdough, pumpernickel or rye bread, whole-wheat or corn tortillas, sandwich or bagel-thins, pretzel buns, pita bread, focaccia, or English muffins.

Include lots of different colors from things like spinach, kale, tomato, onions, cucumber, bell peppers (red, orange, yellow or green), banana peppers, avocado, olives, radishes, shredded carrots or cabbage, beetroot, and bean or alfalfa sprouts.

Include a lean protein like chicken breast, turkey, ham, roast beef, steak, tuna, grilled fish filet, smoked salmon, or egg. Include one slice of cheese like cheddar, provolone, goat cheese, mozzarella, Swiss, Colby-Jack, Gouda, or Muenster.

Stick with condiments like yellow mustard, Dijon mustard, ketchup, light mayo, Sriracha, Tabasco, hummus, avocado/guacamole, light spreadable cheese like Laughing Cow wedges, pesto, vinaigrette, jam, or honey.

And remember, when it comes to packing a lunch, don't underestimate the power of leftovers! If you make extra chicken or whatever healthy protein you're cooking for dinner the night before, you have a ready-made healthy protein option for your sandwich or wrap.

10

GET COOKING

Depending on your upbringing and your college living experience, it's possible that you already know your way around a kitchen, thank you very much. But for many collegiate athletes, cooking is limited largely to microwave meals, frozen pizzas, and mac n' cheese. It's even possible that between the meals provided by your team and athletic department and eating out at cheap joints around campus, you didn't have to do any cooking at all.

As an adult in the real world, learning even some basic cooking skills will benefit both your nutrition goals and your wallet. Relying on restaurants and fast food joints not only racks up calories quickly, it also has a big impact financially.

To put it in perspective, eating out for just two or three meals could easily run you as much as a week's worth of groceries depending on where you're dining. Put that new fancy salary of yours to better use and buy a few basic kitchen essentials and get to cooking. *(Besides, for you single guys and gals, being even a decent cook will only make you an even better catch on the dating scene.)*

Buying kitchen tools and utensils doesn't have to be a big investment, but it is important to at least get the basics, as one of the biggest obstacles for people trying to improve their kitchen skills is that they don't have the necessary tools.

Check out the kitchen essentials below to see where you may need to fill in the gaps.

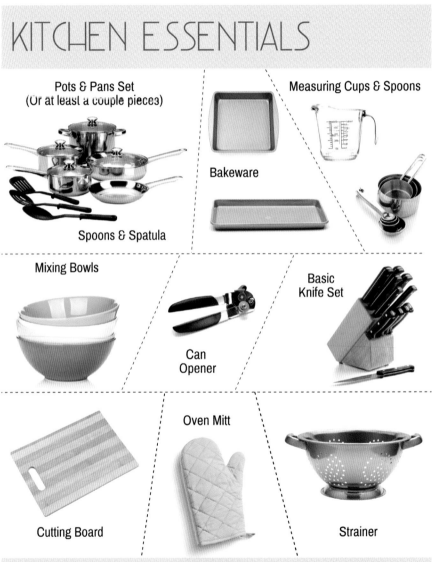

KITCHEN ESSENTIALS

Pots & Pans Set
(Or at least a couple pieces)

Spoons & Spatula

Bakeware

Measuring Cups & Spoons

Mixing Bowls

Can Opener

Basic Knife Set

Oven Mitt

Cutting Board

Strainer

Kitchenware doesn't have to cost a fortune! Many brands have lines that are stylish, yet affordable (see example prices below). If that is still beyond your budget, wait for sales, or try picking up essential pieces at yard sales or at secondhand stores.

Pots & Pans Set - $100, 8" Square Bakeware - $14, Large Nonstick Cookie Sheet - $12, Measuring Cups $15, Measuring Spoons $5, Mixing Bowls $20, Can Opener $12, Knife Set $50, Cutting Board $15, Oven Mitt $7, Strainer $20.

There are a handful of other bonus items that I highly recommend:

Slow cookers (you may know them by the brand name Crock-Pot) are possibly the best invention for ~~lazy~~ busy people ever. You almost have to try to mess up a slow-cooker recipe. Seriously. It usually involves dumping in a handful of ingredients, possibly stirring, plugging it in, and pushing a button. Then you leave for work and come home to deliciousness. You can even put things in frozen, which is even better for ~~lazy~~ busy people. Best part? They're cheap. You can find one for as little as $30!

Rice cookers are less well known, but a true kitchen gem for quickly and easily whipping up a healthy carbohydrate side dish. For those of you thinking, *It cooks rice, so what?!*—rice can actually be tricky to cook, leaving you with anything from dry bits stuck-to the pan to a mushy wet mess. Not to mention some rice grains can take 45 minutes to an hour to cook! A rice cooker speeds up this process and gives you a consistent product each time. Again, you can pick up a smaller one for about $30.

Grills are often thought of as a "man's domain," but male or female, if your living situation allows it, you should consider buying one. Not only are grills easy and quick to use (especially gas or electric ones), but they're a very lean cooking method, because the fat drips off. Even better, they create a delicious product and involve practically no cleanup. What's not to love?! A grill will be a more expensive purchase, but you can get a nice brand for as low as $100 to $300. Cheaper still would be a small portable charcoal or electric grill, which are typically allowed even in apartments . . . although you should definitely check with your landlord before you take my word for it. I don't want the eviction notice taped to your door on my conscience! Even something as simple as an indoor George Foreman grill is better than nothing.

Now you know what you need to get crackin' in the kitchen. If funds are a little tight, consider skipping a weekend of hitting the bars. That should put a little extra spending money in your pocket.

The right tools will go a long way, but now we have to talk about the cooking itself! Really learning to cook is something that happens in the kitchen, not by reading a book, but here are a few tips that can get you started in a healthy direction:

1. **Always keep the basics on hand.**

   This will help you stick to your plan when you haven't been shopping yet, or if your plans change unexpectedly. In the refrigerator: milk, eggs, butter. In the freezer: chicken, ground beef/turkey, veggies. In the pantry: flour, sugar, cooking spray, pasta, bread, rice, cereal, oatmeal, olive oil, spices, salt and pepper.

2. **Don't rely on prepackaged and processed meals.**

   Boxed pasta meals, frozen dinners, and microwave dishes are convenient and fast, but they lack nutritional value and are often loaded with sugar, fat, and sodium.

3. **Start simple.**

   Choose recipes that have short ingredient lists with foods you recognize.

4. **Stick to the recipe.**

   Ingredients, amounts, temperatures, and cooking times were chosen for a reason. As you get more familiar with certain foods and spices, you'll have plenty of opportunity to mix it up a bit and experiment, but until then stick to the recipe and you'll probably be much more satisfied with your end product.

5. **Read the entire recipe before you start.**

   There's nothing more frustrating than getting halfway into making the delicious meal you've been thinking about all day and realizing you're missing an ingredient, or worse, that you've missed a crucial step!

6. **Actually measure stuff.**

   Your recipes will be much more successful, plus measuring is helpful if you're tracking calories or other nutrients. It's easy to misjudge

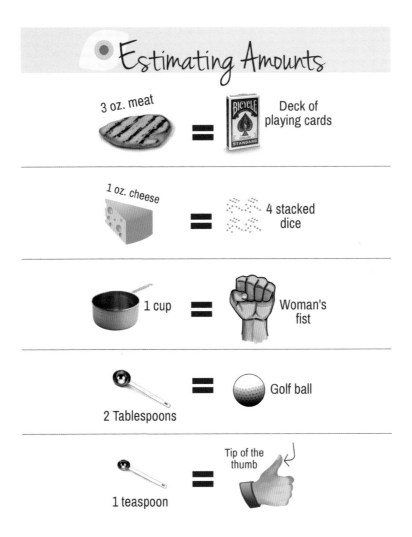

Estimating Amounts

3 oz. meat = Deck of playing cards

1 oz. cheese = 4 stacked dice

1 cup = Woman's fist

2 Tablespoons = Golf ball

1 teaspoon = Tip of the thumb

portion sizes, so actually measure the food a couple of times to get a feel for how much you're really eating. That said, if you're in a pinch, the chart above can help you make smart estimates.

7. **Don't rely on salt to make things taste better.**

I've mentioned sodium (aka salt) here and there, but we haven't really talked about Normal Human sodium intake yet. For athletes, sodium isn't often a nutrient that we're concerned about. In fact, if it is, it's usually because we're concerned about not getting enough. As a Normal Human, this is no longer the case. Athletes need sodium in higher amounts because they lose it in their sweat. But for the more recreational exerciser, it's unlikely that conditions will promote extreme sweating.

The 2015–2020 Dietary Guidelines recommend that Americans consume less than 2,300 mg of sodium per day as part of a healthy eating pattern. Sounds like a lot, right? Wrong. Most Americans consume well over this recommendation, often doubling or tripling the amount. Why does that matter? Excess sodium increases your blood pressure, which creates an added burden for your heart. Over time, too much sodium in your diet increases the risk of heart disease, stroke, and certain cancers, to name a few.

If you're thinking, *Fine, bossy lady, I'll just quit salting my food*, it's actually not that easy. While reducing table salt is a good place to start, most of the sodium in our diets comes from processed foods and the amounts add up quickly. To keep your sodium consumption in check, try limiting the following foods in your Normal Human diet: canned foods like soup, deli meat and cheese, processed meats like salami, bacon, and sausage, snack foods like chips and crackers, boxed pasta and rice meals, and certain sauces and salad dressings. In addition to limiting those foods, you can also look for low-sodium canned options, which are becoming more common. You can also rinse canned vegetables with water to reduce sodium.

If you're someone who relies on salt to flavor your food, try flavoring dishes with things like lemon or lime, garlic, onion, pepper, and other herbs and spices. Sodium is listed on food labels, so especially when it comes to prepackaged foods, glance at the label to find out if it's loaded with sneaky sodium.

8. **Keep your food safe**

   Some important rules to live by to avoid food poisoning:

   ✓ If you touch raw meat, immediately wash your hands before touching other food.

   ✓ Don't use cutting boards, knives, or other utensils that were used with raw meat on anything else.

   ✓ Wash fruits and vegetables.

   ✓ Cook meat to safe internal temperatures.

   ✓ If you have any doubts, this is another great opportunity to put your smartphone to work. Download the "Is My Food Safe?" app and ask away.

9. **Cook in batches**

   Make more than you'll need for just that one meal. Leftovers are perfect for packing your lunch or an easy solution for nights you're in a rush and don't have time to cook. Depending on the meal,

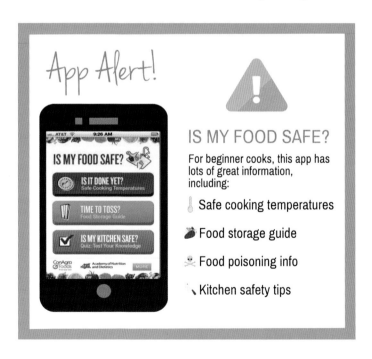

the leftovers can even be frozen. Soups, casseroles, and pasta dishes make for great freezer-friendly leftovers.

10. **Prep ahead of time**

Just like cooking in batches, this step can save you time and stress in the long run. Pick one night each week that you can chop up some fruit/veggies or trim some meat.

11. **Use your resources**

You live in an age where anything and everything is available online at the click of a button: endless recipes, countless cooking tips, and life hacks. Wondering how to cut an onion? How to tell if your salmon is cooked? Google it. You're guaranteed to find a picture tutorial and video on the subject.

11

REDEFINING YOURSELF

The last part of this book I write not as a sports dietitian, but as someone who has made the transition from athlete to Normal Human and watched countless friends and student athletes do so as well. Just as you've had to work to figure out what your diet and workout plan should be as a Normal Human, most athletes find there is a mental aspect of the transition as well.

One of the hardest parts of this transition for many athletes is that they have formed much of their self-identity around their sport. Sport-specific training now starts at an incredibly young age, and many athletes pour hours of their childhood into perfecting technique, building endurance and learning the game—sometimes leaving little time for developing other talents. You may have found that you missed out on some things that your nonathlete peers considered a part of a "normal childhood"—such as getting a job, going on school trips, and having sleepovers.

As a retired athlete, you will find (or may have already found) that one day, after all those years of training, it just ends. For many it ends rather abruptly. It's a moment that you've always known would come, but that doesn't stop the whirlwind of emotions you're left to deal with after the last whistle blows. Sadness. Panic. Maybe relief. Usually confusion over what to do next.

A life that has always been filled with a tightly dictated schedule of practices, meetings, weight lifting sessions, and conditioning suddenly opens up.

From the blog . . .

August?

It may sound strange, but as a collegiate athlete playing a fall sport, August is a mythical legend . . . a month only enjoyed by people far removed from the grind of college sports. A typical summer for an athlete may involve a short time off to recover and relax, but then it's right back to campus to work out with your team and take a few summer classes to lighten the load during the school year.

By the time mid-July rolls around, you can expect full-fledged panic to have set in, as preseason draws closer and closer. Between the fitness tests, meetings, sleeping, and the overall stress that preseason brings, August pretty much flies by. Then you wake up one morning, camp is over, and you're starting classes.

So here I am, August 8th, sitting in a local café, feeling super normal wondering, *What do Normal Humans do during this month?!* The obvious answer is work I suppose . . . but for recent "retirees" like myself, for instance, who are waiting for internships to start? I'm at a loss.

I did however, recently partake in playing 11 vs. 11 with the current team, which is low on numbers due to injuries. If that doesn't slap you into realization of how old and out of shape you are, I don't know what will. After the first 15 minutes of playing I think I was hindering my team more than helping them. I woke up this morning and every join and muscle on my body hurt, aside from maybe my fingers.

While I certainly miss the preseason bonding time with my teammates, given the physical exhaustion and pain, paired with the fact that you're trapped in a hotel most of the month, I have to give the month of August to Normal Humanhood. Now I just have to figure out what to do with it. Currently accepting friendship applications via email, Facebook, and postal services . . .

What will you do tomorrow when you don't have to report to the team meeting? What will you do every afternoon when you've always had practice? It is this realization that leaves many athletes thinking, *If I don't have my sport, what* do *I have?*

This is a question that only you can answer, but I encourage you to have an open mind about it, because you are so much more than just your sport.

Don't think about the door that's closing on your sport. Focus instead on what a fantastic experience you had—and the countless doors to opportunities your sport has opened for you.

You hopefully have a great degree in hand that you can use to continue to open more doors. You've made connections throughout your state, and likely throughout the country. Connect with people in that network and use it to your advantage.

Your sport does not define you, but it has helped to define how you will handle future situations. It has taught you discipline, commitment, time management, and teamwork, and it has shown you the joy of success and the heartbreak of defeat. Remember that. These are all things that will make you a successful Normal Human. Not to mention qualities that employers value!

So what *will* define you? Hopefully not just one thing. Maybe it will be your career. Your family and friends. Maybe you will find new talents, or rekindle old ones long forgotten during your athletic career. Perhaps you have a passion for cooking, traveling, or music, to name a few. Explore the passions you haven't had time for as an athlete.

For some of you, your sport may continue to play an important role in your life through coaching, mentoring, intramural leagues, and pickup games, or even officiating. Whether it does or not, remember fondly your "glory days" and set out to redefine yourself—Normal Human style! The more prepared you are for this change, and the more acceptance you have regarding it, the happier you will be.

12

GOING IT ALONE

Another common hurdle retired athletes encounter is loneliness. The rigorous demands of college athletics mean that you spend much of your time with your teammates. There's no getting around it. Love them or hate them, you will know your teammates as well as your family by the time you graduate. Your team has provided a constant social circle for the last four or five years.

In my own experience, my college teammates were my best friends, and we did everything together. Everything. Even when we stepped off the soccer field, we ate together, drank together, lived together . . . It's a wonder we managed to still like each other after so many years in such close quarters!

One of the very real struggles of Normal Humanhood is that after graduation, pretty much everyone leaves, either to go back to their hometown or off to new cities for new jobs and new adventures. Before you know it, the girls or guys you've spent every waking moment with over the last 4 to 5 years are scattered around the country or globe.

It can be a hard reality to accept. So hard, that maybe at first you find yourself sulking at home, looking through old Facebook albums thinking, *Take me back!* But then you think, *I'm a fun person, I'm outgoing! This is no big deal. I'm going to go make some new friends!*

From the blog . . .

You get by with a little help from your friends

If I had to pick the one worst thing about no longer being an athlete, it would absolutely be that I'm no longer surrounded by my teammates all the time.

Anyone who's been a part of a team on any level would probably agree that one of the best parts about it is the bond you share with your teammates. Even more so when you take your sport to the collegiate level, because you do *everything* together. From that terrifying moment your parents drop you off at preseason freshman year, you become completely immersed in the program, all up in each others' biz-nazz 24/7.

You live in a hotel with your teammates for a month before anyone else is even on campus. You move into the dorms with each other as freshmen. You find houses to live in together as sophomores. You eat, sleep, and party together. You come back during the summers when campus is empty so you can train together. Maybe more than anything else, you endure awful workouts together and often you only get through them because you know the girl next to you will kick your ass if she has to do one more rerun because you didn't make it.

While this process creates lifetime bonds, it does have one downfall: You spend all of your time with other student athletes. So now that I'm done, am I just expected to meet new people on my own?! Preposterous. They won't understand the pain of running Ross Ade Stadium, or doing sand workouts. They probably won't think I'm even speaking English if I mention Mollenkopf Athletic Center! What will we even talk about?!

For the moment I'm going to cling to the fact that I still live on campus and have access to my teammates, but I can't say that I'm excited for the many future, potentially awkward conversations I'm bound to have with other Normal Humans . . .

Sometimes this works great, and sometimes it's harder than you think. You may luck out and land a job with lots of young coworkers in a happenin' city with great nightlife. Or you may find that your new office is comprised of mostly middle-aged adults who race off to pick up their kids after work, or that the bar scene in your new city is a far cry from the one you loved in college.

Regardless of what situation you're in, you may also find that you're not really "clicking" with anyone. After all, your whole life has been spent surrounded by teammates. You effortlessly had an immediate group of friends who were your age and shared similar interests—certainly at least one similar interest!

Making friends in the real world can feel a lot like dating. Wondering if they like you back . . . wanting to ask them to hang out but with the looming fear of rejection. The good news is that they're probably thinking the same thing. So what can you do to build up a new network of friends?

1. Don't be intimidated. If you feel like the people you've met aren't super friendly, remember that people may find you intimidating. After all, you're young, have "collegiate athlete" on your résumé, and of course you're following my advice so you look great!

2. Reach out! Don't be afraid to ask new coworkers to grab a drink after work (*this is a good reason to break your workweek no-alcohol rule*). If your coworkers aren't a group you see yourself meshing with, reach out to others. Remember those tips about meeting people who share your workout interests? Playing on an intramural team or being part of a group fitness class can be a perfect place to meet people with similar interests.

3. Get out in the community. It's easy to fall into your routine and put "Get involved" at the bottom of your to-do list, but this is another great avenue for meeting people with similar interests and networking within your community. If you're religious, get involved with a religious institution such as a local church, synagogue, or temple. If you're passionate about a cause, find a local organization dedicated to it. Go cuddle the cats and dogs at your local animal shelter.

Athlete case files

In another excerpt from my own file, my husband (a former collegiate football player turned Normal Human) and I had been living in our house for about a year when some new neighbors moved in next door.

During a short conversation on the lawn they seemed really great—they were our age and planned to stay for a while. We were really excited at the idea of having neighbors that we could hang out with, but we were nervous. Did we have the same interests? Would we actually get along? Maybe they would think we were annoying or weird, or maybe they had no interest in getting to know us.

For the first couple months after they moved in we debated inviting them to do something, but kept chickening out. It felt like trying to work up the courage to ask someone to the middle school dance. Instead of just marching over and inviting them to have dinner, we silently creeped on them for a while. We would look out the window and discover, "Oh! They're grilling out. . . . *We* like to grill out!" or "Ooh look, they're having a beer. . . . *We* enjoy a good brew now and then!"

These discoveries gave us enough good vibes to finally muster up the courage to ask them to join us for a cookout, annnnd they were busy. We thought, *Crap. We were right. They don't want to hang out with us.* Looking back, it all sounds ridiculous because we DID eventually have the chance to hang out and they're now great friends of ours.

As we got to know them better, they admitted they were doing the same things—trying to catch a glimpse of what we were up to, wondering if they should ask us to do something, and being nervous that we might be put off by the idea. Luckily we didn't waste too much time being creepy window neighbors, or we would have missed out on a great opportunity to make new friends.

4. Use your alumni network. Every university has at least some sort of alumni group and network—reach out to them and find out what other alumni are in your area and whether there are any upcoming events. They may not be former athletes, but you certainly share a common interest in your alma mater.

5. Stay in touch. Even though you'll meet lots of great new people, don't neglect the ones you were so distraught over leaving after college. It's easy to slip into the trap of following your friends' lives on Facebook and feeling like you're staying in touch without really talking. Call or text old friends when you have the chance. Schedule trips to see each other, especially while you're young and have fewer financial commitments—and before everyone starts having babies n' stuff.

Most importantly, don't beat yourself up if it's taking a while for you to make new friends. That's another totally Normal Human experience. And if your loneliness starts to feel overwhelming, don't be embarrassed to seek out a counselor to talk things over.

When it's all said and done, being an athlete will always be a part of who you are, but it is not all of who you are. Embrace this new Normal Human chapter of your life and set out to find what else you can bring to the table.

CONCLUSION

All in all, life as a Normal Human has been a lot of things for me. Weird. Sad. Exciting. New.

Most likely, it will be a mix of things for you, too. Your transition to Normal Humanhood and your reactions to it may be similar to those of your teammates, but they could very well be entirely different. Just like everyone's experience as an athlete is different, so is everyone's experience as a Normal Human.

You may find a new sport or activity that you love right away and find that you're rocking it in the kitchen but really struggling to meet people with interests similar to yours. Meanwhile, your closest teammate and friend might have a great new group of friends but have a difficult time balancing energy needs and finding a new exercise niche in his/her new lifestyle. Lean on your teammates and friends and help each other adjust.

The good news is that you've taken a great first step in reading this book. Even if you decide that you want nothing to do with my nutrition and fitness advice, one of the most important things you can do to prepare for Normal Humanhood is just to acknowledge that it's coming—or for some of you, that it's here. It's easy to pretend otherwise, to just push the thoughts of your impending new lifestyle far, far away and to keep clinging to your identity as an athlete that you've always known. While plenty of people take this approach, it almost always catches up to them. Usually, the longer they've waited to acknowledge their new reality, the harder it is to adjust when they finally have to.

While your days as an athlete will always be a part of you, they do not define you. When times seem tough, think back to all of the skills you gained from your experience as an athlete. Time management. Overcoming adversity. Resiliency. Teamwork and leadership. And so many more. These are all attributes that will make you a successful employee, spouse, parent, and friend.

If I had to summarize my advice in just a few bullet points, it would boil down to this:

1. **Strive for balance—in all aspects of your life.**
   Balance those fun foods with healthy foods. Vary your workouts to include cardio, strengthening, and just-for-fun activities. Make sure work doesn't overtake your life. Make time for friends and family . . . and for yourself!

2. **Forget perfection.**
   As athletes we were trained to aim for perfection. Keep doing the drill until you get it just right. As students we were told that our GPA couldn't be high enough if we wanted to be competitive for that dream job. But the truth is, the real world is far from perfect. And your nutrition and fitness plan certainly won't be perfect either. At the end of the day, don't beat yourself up when things don't go as planned. Use that resiliency you've learned, pick yourself back up, and try again. Sometimes mistakes and shortfalls lead to the best experiences.

3. **Stay connected.**
   As I mentioned in the last chapter, it's easy to get caught up with your busy new life. In the age of texting, Snapchat, and social media it's easy to feel like you're staying in touch while actually falling *out* of touch with old friends. Make time to visit your old teammates, get home to visit family, and make the occasional trip back to your alma mater to see what things have changed and soak in the things that haven't. You'll never regret picking up the phone and calling an old friend or visiting the new city they've moved to. Life only gets busier!

4. **Seek professional help if needed.**

Reading a book is great, and I truly hope that mine has helped you as you're entering this new phase of your life, but if certain aspects of the transition are extra difficult or feel out of control, seek help sooner than later. As I've mentioned multiple times, make sure that help is coming from a credentialed professional, not some guru practicing out of their van (okay, dramatic, but you know what I mean). Whether it's a dietitian, certified personal trainer, psychologist, or otherwise, they can be a huge help if something feels too hard to manage on your own.

So there you have it, my best advice in a book-sized nutshell on living your best Normal Human life. Best of luck to you; now go do the damn thing!

APPENDIX A: RECIPES FOR BEGINNERS

OVERNIGHT OATS

This tasty cold breakfast option is a great meal to prep a few of at a time, since they last a few days in the fridge and are perfect when you're running late and need a grab n' go option on your way out the door!

They're also very versatile, which I think you'll see as you read on.

Base Ingredients:

(Per one serving)
- ¼ cup old fashioned oats, dry
- ¼ cup vanilla Greek yogurt
- ⅓ cup skim or 2% milk
- 2 Tbsp. chia seeds

Additional ingredients

Fruit and whatever the heck else you want to put in it. This can really be anything from fresh, dried, or frozen fruit, nuts or nut butters, vanilla, cocoa, and everything in between!

A few of my favorite combos include:

- Fresh berries and 1 Tbsp. almond butter
- Dried cherries and 1 tsp. vanilla extract
- Sliced banana and 1 Tbsp. peanut butter

Directions

1. Combine all base ingredients in reusable plastic or glass container and stir to mix
2. Add desired additional ingredients to taste
3. Store in refrigerator overnight and eat cold the next day or over the next week

EGG MUFFINS

These are essentially baby omelets, and are another great option when you need a to-go breakfast option—they can keep in the fridge for up to a week, or can be frozen.

Ingredients

- Cooking spray
- ½ cup veggies of choice, finely chopped (I recommend bell pepper, onion, and mushroom)
- 1 dozen large eggs (may also use just egg whites, but you'll need more eggs to fill your muffin tin cups)
- ½ cup meat of choice, cooked (I recommend breakfast sausage, ham, or turkey)

Directions

1. Preheat oven to 350
2. Spray muffin tin with cooking spray
3. Divide veggies and meat evenly among the holes in the muffin tin
4. Whisk together eggs in a medium bowl until the yolk and whites are well combined and add evenly to each muffin tin cup. Each hole should be about ⅔ full.
5. Bake at 350 for about 10 minutes. The egg muffins should rise to fill the cup up, and should be just a little golden on top.
6. May be eaten immediately, or refrigerated or frozen to eat later on!

   If they're coming from the fridge, 1 minute in the microwave should be sufficient to heat them up. I suggest sprinkling a little shredded cheese on top, and either eating plain, or flattening one or two of them between toast or an English muffin to make a quick sandwich!

JUDY KAY'S CHILI

My dear mother's super-secret (until now) chili recipe. Stupid easy and delicious and can even be done in a slow cooker. I recommend making at least a double batch.

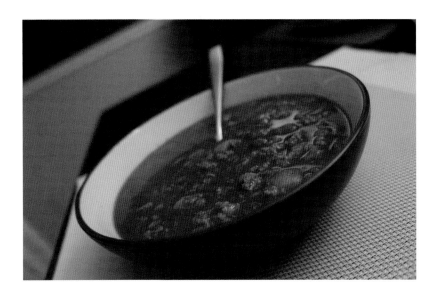

Ingredients

- 1 lb. ground beef (or ground turkey)
- 1 medium onion, chopped
- 15 oz. tomato sauce
- 1 can (15 oz.) hot chili beans
- 1 cup water
- 1 tsp. salt
- 1 tsp. chili powder
- Pepper, to taste
- 1 bay leaf

Directions

1. Brown ground beef (or turkey) and onion.
2. Add rest of ingredients.
3. Cook covered on low for 1 hour, stirring occasionally.

SIMPLE TERIYAKI STIR-FRY

My go-to easy recipe when I've got some veggies that are about to be past their prime!

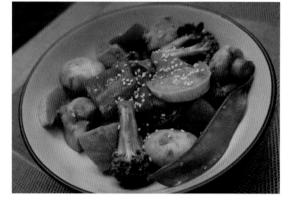

Ingredients

Teriyaki Sauce

- ¼ cup soy sauce
- ¼ cup water
- 1 Tbsp. brown sugar
- 1 tsp. chopped ginger
- 1 tsp. crushed garlic
- ¼ cup minced onion

In a pinch you can substitute a store-bought teriyaki sauce but be aware that it may be higher in sugar content.

Stir-Fry

- 1 lb. chicken or steak, cubed (about 1 inch)
- Any and all veggies (my favorites: chopped bell peppers, snow peas, chopped onion, broccoli florets, chopped zucchini)

Directions

1. Add all sauce ingredients to a small mixing bowl and whisk together until combined.
2. In a large heated skillet or wok, add meat and sauce, stirring often for 5 minutes. For stronger flavor allow meat to marinate, refrigerated in teriyaki sauce for at least 2–3 hours.
3. Add veggies in and stir often, for 10–15 minutes or until veggies are tender enough to easily pierce with a fork, but not mushy.
4. Serve over brown rice for a balanced meal!

CHICKEN À LA CROCK-POT

It's actually stupid to even call this a recipe.

Ingredients

- 2–4 pounds chicken breasts
- ½ cup water
- Salt
- Pepper

Directions

1. Trim any visible fat off the chicken.
2. Place chicken into slow cooker with the water.
3. Sprinkle with salt and pepper.
4. Close lid and turn the slow cooker on low-medium for 6 to 8 hours.

FAKED POTATO

Because baking a potato in the oven takes like, forever . . . give or take.

Ingredients

- 1 Potato

Directions

1. Using a fork, poke a few holes in the washed potato.
2. Place potato in microwave and microwave for 6 to 7 minutes, or until soft. Alternatively, if your microwave has a "potato" button—push it.

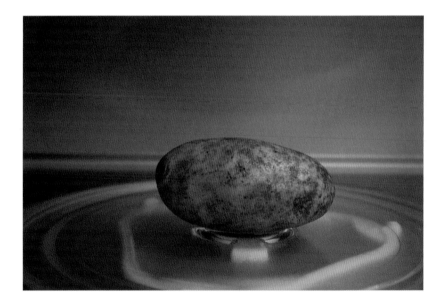

ROASTED ASPARAGUS

Delicious and versatile side. Note: Asparagus will make your pee smell weird. Don't panic, it's normal.

Ingredients

- 1 bunch asparagus
- 2 Tbsp. olive oil
- Salt and pepper to taste

Directions

1. Preheat oven to 350 degrees.
2. Wash and cut stems off asparagus.
3. Lay stalks side by side on greased baking sheet and drizzle with olive oil.
4. Sprinkle with salt and pepper.
5. Bake for 10 to 15 minutes or until they can be easily pierced with a fork.

Try drizzling balsamic vinegar over the asparagus for a sweet and tangy twist!

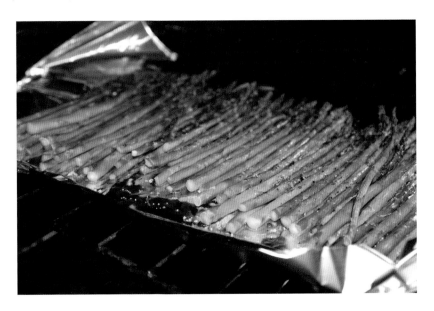

BORING BROCCOLI

Boring . . . but easy!

Ingredients

¼ cup water
3–4 cups broccoli florets

Directions

1. Pour water into a large microwave-safe container. It should cover just the bottom.
2. Add broccoli florets, and cover container loosely with lid.
3. Microwave for 4 to 5 minutes or until broccoli is tender.

ROASTED BROCCOLI

Broccoli doesn't have to be boring!

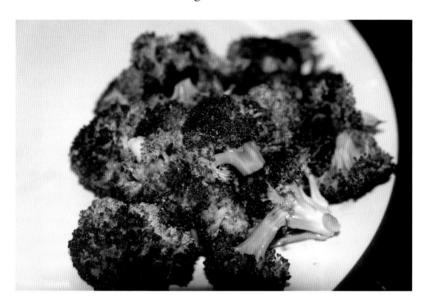

Ingredients

- 3–4 cups broccoli florets
- ¼ cup olive oil
- 1 Tbsp. minced garlic

Directions

1. Preheat oven to 425.
2. In large mixing bowl, toss broccoli with olive oil and garlic.
3. Spread broccoli evenly across baking sheet and bake for 15–20 minutes until crispy and easily pierced with a fork.

STOP! IT'S SALMON THYME

Don't let cooking fish intimidate you. This simple recipe is great for beginner cooks and will have you eating those yummy omega-3s before you know it!

Ingredients

- 1 or 2 salmon fillets, thawed
- 1 Tbsp. olive oil
- 2 Tbsp. lemon juice, preferably fresh
- 1 tsp. rosemary
- 1 tsp. thyme
- 1 pinch salt

Directions

1. Preheat oven to 375°.
2. Take large piece of foil and place salmon inside it.
3. Drizzle with olive oil and lemon juice and sprinkle with rosemary, thyme, and salt.
4. Wrap foil up around salmon loosely, but close tightly at top.
5. Bake for 15 to 20 minutes. Salmon should be opaque and flake apart with a fork.

SPICY TACO SKILLET

Versatile, delicious, and takes one pan. Oh, and it sneaks in lots of veggies!

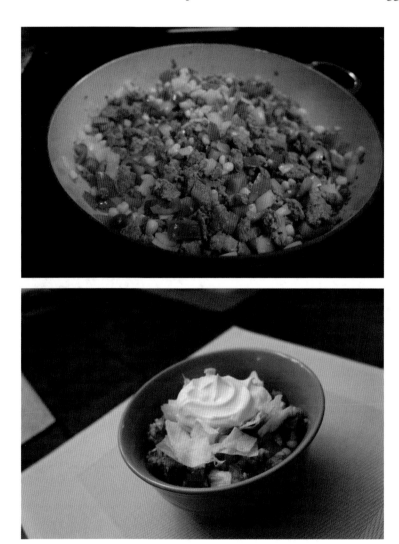

Ingredients

- 1 pound ground turkey or beef
- 1 large onion, diced
- 1 bell pepper, diced

- 1 cup corn, frozen or canned
- 1 15-oz. can of diced tomatoes and green chilies
- 1 cup salsa
- 1 cup rice or orzo (I prefer orzo)
- 1 cup water
- 1 cup chicken or beef broth
- 2 tsp. cumin*
- ½ tsp. cayenne pepper*
- 1 tsp. chili powder*
- 1 tsp. garlic powder*
- 1 tsp. smoked paprika*
- 1 cup shredded cheddar or jack cheese
- 1 cup shredded lettuce (optional)
- Sour cream (optional)

Directions

1. In a large pan, brown turkey or beef.
2. When ground meat is lightly browned, add diced onion and pepper.
3. Cook until beef is fully cooked, and onions and peppers are soft.
4. Add corn and can of diced tomatoes and green chilies—no need to drain.
5. Add salsa, rice/orzo, water, and broth.
6. Stir well to combine.
7. Add in spices and mix, cover.
8. Let simmer on low until rice is soft and liquid has cooked off, about 20–30 minutes.
9. Top with cheese, stirring in until it melts. Serve with shredded lettuce and sour cream if desired!

If you don't have all of these spices, replace all spices listed with 1 packet of taco seasoning.

CHICKEN AND CORN CHOWDER

Great for chilly weather, and loaded with sneaky veggies!

Ingredients

- 2 Tbsp. olive oil
- 1 medium onion, diced
- 1 cup celery, diced
- ¼ tsp. cayenne pepper
- 1 tsp. dried oregano
- ¼ tsp. salt
- ¼ cup flour
- 4 cups chicken or vegetable broth
- 2 cups yellow summer squash, diced
- 2 cups sweet potato, diced
- 2 cups fresh corn kernels
- 1 red bell pepper, diced
- 3 or 4 chicken breasts, cooked and cubed or shredded

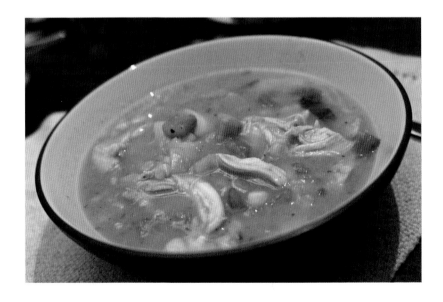

Directions

1. In a large pan, heat the oil over medium heat.
2. Add the onion and celery and cook until softened, about 5 minutes.
3. Add the cayenne pepper, oregano, and salt and stir together. Sprinkle the flour over the onion and celery and stir constantly for 1 minute until the flour starts to brown and coat the vegetables.
4. Whisk in the broth and bring to a boil.
5. Reduce the heat to low and add the remaining ingredients: squash, sweet potato, corn, and bell pepper.
6. Stirring occasionally, simmer for an additional 15 minutes until the vegetables are tender.
7. Ladle 2 cups of vegetables into a blender or food processor, pouring out as much broth as possible. Puree the vegetables in a blender until smooth.
8. Add the pureed vegetables back into the pot and stir together. Add the cooked, shredded chicken and mix in. Cook for an additional 5 minutes until thickened.
9. Serve and top with garnishes such as sour cream, cilantro, or shredded cheese if desired.

LINKO DE MAYO ENCHILADAS

My husband and I started dating on Cinco de Mayo (romantic, I know) . . . and even though we have a new anniversary now we vowed to always commemorate our original anniversary with delicious enchiladas and margaritas. Here's my recipe.

Ingredients

- 1 lb. ground beef OR shredded chicken (great use of Crock-Pot chicken recipe, or can use canned chicken)
- 1 small onion, chopped
- 1 bell pepper (any color), chopped
- 1 jalapeño, chopped (optional)
- 1 can diced tomatoes and green chilies, drained
- ¼ cup fresh cilantro, chopped
- The juice of 1 lime (or 4 Tbsp. of lime juice)
- 1 tsp. cumin
- 1 tsp. chili powder
- 1 tsp. minced garlic
- 1 package of whole-wheat tortillas—8–10
- 1 can of red enchilada sauce
- 1 cup shredded Colby Jack cheese

Directions

1. Preheat oven to 350°.
2. Add beef to large skillet and cook over medium-high heat until brown, drain off fat. If using chicken, add cooked, shredded chicken to skillet.
3. Add chopped onion, pepper, and jalapeño. Cook until soft and translucent, about 5 minutes.
4. Drain diced tomatoes and green chilies and add to skillet.
5. Add cilantro, lime juice, cumin, chili powder, and garlic and stir to combine. Cook another 2–3 minutes.

6. Take skillet off heat and prep enchiladas.
7. Spray 9 × 13 pan with cooking spray
8. Take 1 tortilla and lay flat on clean counter surface. Spoon about ½ cup of enchilada filling into shell. Fold shell in half—away from your body. Fold both ends in toward the center and roll into a cylinder. Place in greased pan.
9. Do this for remaining tortillas, or until you run out of filling. Place enchiladas closely together in pan; fit as many as needed into pan by squishing together if needed.
10. Pour can of enchilada sauce over the top of enchiladas, attempting to cover as much as possible.
11. Sprinkle cheese over enchiladas and place in oven.
12. Cook uncovered until bubbly—about 15 minutes.
13. Serve with shredded lettuce, tomato, avocado, salsa, sour cream, pickled jalapeño, and anything else that tickles your fancy.

VEGGIE MARINADE

This simple veggie marinade that our neighbors introduced us to is easy and seriously clutch for that quick last-minute side that you need to supply for the cookout! It's also a tasty way to use up those veggies that are about to go bad!

Ingredients

- Any and all chopped veggies (I suggest zucchini/squash, peppers, onion, mushrooms, and Brussels sprouts)
- ½ cup reduced sodium soy sauce
- ½ cup water
- 2 Tbsp. minced garlic
- 1 Tbsp. cumin

Directions

1. Chop all veggies so they are a similar size
2. Add to large bowl or freezer-sized plastic bag
3. Add remaining ingredients, and stir
4. Let sit for at least 30 minutes, or up to 3–4 hours
5. Cook on the grill—in a grill basket or on aluminum foil until veggies are easily pierced with a fork and look crispy from the grill

FRENCH DIP SAMMICHES

This is a simple but delicious meal, and is a different way to include red meat in your diet and get all those beneficial B vitamins and iron!

Ingredients

- 1 can of beef broth/stock
- 1 Tbsp. Worchestershire sauce
- 1 tsp. garlic powder
- Black pepper, to taste
- 1 lb. deli roast beef, shaved or thinly sliced
- 1 fresh baguette
- ¼ lb. sliced provolone cheese

Directions

1. Heat beef broth, Worchestershire sauce, garlic powder, and black pepper over medium pot
2. Once broth is warm, add roast beef to pot to heat up, about 5–10 minutes
3. While roast beef is heating up, cut baguette into 6–8-inch pieces, and slice each in half
4. Toast baguette pieces in oven or toaster until lightly browned
5. Using tongs, put 4–5 oz. of roast beef on each half baguette, and top with a slice of provolone cheese. Complete the sandwich by putting the other half of the baguette on top
6. Ladle about ½ cup of the broth into a small bowl for dipping the sandwich into
7. Serve sandwich with small broth bowl for dipping, along with a side salad or veggie

GRILLED/SAUTÉED SHRIMP

Shrimp are actually a great lean protein source that only take minutes (literally, single-digit minutes) to cook!

Ingredients

- ¼ cup olive oil
- Juice from 1 lime (about 4 Tbsp.)
- 1 tsp. red pepper flakes
- 1 tsp. minced garlic
- 1 pinch paprika
- Large raw deveined, thawed shrimp (About 12 to 15 shrimp, serves 2 people)

Directions

1. Add all ingredients except the shrimp to a medium bowl and mix together
2. Add shrimp and toss in the mixture
3. In a skillet or on foil over the grill, add shrimp and cook for about 3 minutes on each side

---

Cooked shrimp will be opaque and a pinkish/white color

APPENDIX B: TIPS FOR HEALTHY WEIGHT GAIN

1. **Follow through** with your workout plan. A well-rounded weight-lifting regimen is key when it comes to building muscle.
2. **Support your training with a high-energy (aka high-calorie) diet** that maintains balance between protein and carbohydrate.

    Protein is key for building muscle, but remember that we can only use 20 to 30 grams at one time for muscle synthesis. Be sure to include protein in moderate amounts at each meal and snack.

    Carbohydrate is often neglected when it comes to building muscle, but it plays an important role. Adequate amounts of carbohydrates will help provide enough calories to support muscle growth.
3. **Eat and drink frequently**—you cannot afford to miss a meal! Aim to eat a meal or a snack every 3 to 4 hours, rather than just increasing the size of your three main meals. This will help increase overall calories and promote muscle growth.
4. **Include healthy foods that are energy-dense.** This means that they have a lot of calories in a small amount of food. These can help bump up your calories without adding a lot of bulk to your diet, which can fill you up quickly. Nuts, nut butters, seeds, trail mix, avocado, guacamole, olive oil, dried fruit, granola, cheese, and coconut are great energy-dense options.
5. **Include healthy beverages that are energy-dense.** By including a beverage that has healthy calories with each meal, you can increase

your calories further without filling up as quickly. Milk, chocolate milk, 100% fruit juice, smoothies, and protein shakes like Ensure or Boost are great energy-dense options.

6. **Maintain consistency.** It will take commitment and planning to ensure that you're not missing meals and that you're including the necessary foods throughout the day, *every day*. If you follow these tips only a few days of the week, you aren't likely to see the results you want.

7. **Seek qualified advice before taking supplements**. As we've discussed, any product with a "Supplements Facts" label is not well regulated, and therefore it is hard to know whether it is safe and effective. Do not turn to the unqualified employee at GNC, your bro at the gym, or blogs to determine whether you need a supplement and which one you should choose. It is very rare that you cannot meet your needs through food.

8. **Monitor progress and adjust when necessary**. Weigh yourself only once a week and try to do it on the same day of the week around the same time of day. A safe rate of weight gain is about 1 to 2 pounds/week, but don't get frustrated if you don't see that gain every single week. Oftentimes you may plateau and need to adjust your plan slightly to continue to see results. Avoid weigh-ins post-workout when you may have lost water weight through sweat that will come right back when you rehydrate.

Energy-dense

Energy density is the amount of energy, or calories, per gram of food. Less-energy-dense foods provide fewer calories per gram of food so you can eat more without consuming as many calories.

Example: 1 cup of carrots has 50 calories. 1 cup of almonds has 800 calories. The almonds would be the more energy-dense option.

Nutrient-dense

Nutrient-dense foods are foods that are high in nutrients (vitamins, minerals, healthy fats, lean protein, complex carbohydrates), but are relatively low in calories.

Example: 1 cup of spinach is high in vitamins E, A, and K and has 7 calories. 1 cup of ice cream has 300 calories and is high in refined sugar and fat. The spinach would be the more nutrient-dense option.

APPENDIX C: TIPS FOR HEALTHY WEIGHT LOSS

1. **Follow through** with your workout plan. Having a consistently higher energy expenditure will help speed up your metabolism and help promote weight loss.
2. **Strive for a nutrient-dense diet** that provides plenty of fruits and vegetables, adequate protein, and moderate amounts of carbohydrate.
   - ✓ **Choose lean options** within each group. Try to fill up on healthy, lean options so that you're not as hungry for options that won't support your goals.
   - ✓ **Limit high-fat options.** While you can certainly include these foods from time to time, limiting them will increase your chances for success. Foods to limit include ribs, wings, bacon, sausage, pepperoni, salami, French fries, breaded or fried foods, hash browns, pizza, butter, sour cream, ranch dressing, and Alfredo sauce.
3. **Eat and drink frequently**! Aim to eat a meal or a snack every 3 to 4 hours. Losing weight does not mean you should be hungry. Skipping meals can slow down your metabolism and lead to overeating at the next meal or snack.
4. **Limit amounts of healthy foods that are energy-dense.** These foods have great health benefits and are nice options to include in your diet. However, their calories can add up quickly, so ensure

that you're moderating the amount that you're consuming when it comes to these foods.

✓ Nuts, nut butters, seeds, trail mix, avocado, guacamole, olive oil, dried fruit, granola, cheese, and coconut offer great nutrition and help satisfy hunger, but they are also energy-dense.

5. **Limit beverages that are energy-dense.** Beverages are an easy way to rack up calories without filling up. Stick to water and other low-calorie choices as much as possible. See page 54 for recommendations.

6. **Maintain consistency.** It will take commitment and planning to ensure that you're not missing meals and that you're including the necessary foods throughout the day, every day. If you follow these tips only a few days a week, you aren't likely to see the results you want.

7. **Seek qualified advice before taking supplements**. As we've discussed, any product with a "Supplements Facts" label is not well regulated, and therefore it is very hard to know whether it is safe and effective. Do not turn to TV shows, magazines, or the Internet to get advice on weight loss. Usually these suggestions are unrealistic and can be unsafe.

8. **Monitor progress and adjust when necessary**. Weigh yourself only once a week and try to do it on the same day of the week around the same time of day. A safe rate of weight loss is about 1 to 2 pounds/week, but don't get frustrated if you don't see that rate every single week. Oftentimes you may plateau and need to adjust your plan slightly to continue to see results.

Energy-dense

Energy density is the amount of energy, or calories, per gram of food. Less-energy-dense foods provide fewer calories per gram of food so you can eat more without consuming as many calories.

Example: 1 cup of carrots has 50 calories. 1 cup of almonds has 800 calories. The almonds would be the more energy-dense option.

Nutrient-dense

Nutrient-dense foods are foods that are high in nutrients (vitamins, minerals, healthy fats, lean protein, complex carbohydrates), but are relatively low in calories.

Example: 1 cup of spinach is high in vitamins E, A, and K and has 7 calories. 1 cup of ice cream has 300 calories and is high in refined sugar and fat. The spinach would be the more nutrient-dense option.

Caution: We live in a dieting-crazed culture—one that is pumping out books and products faster than the public can keep up! Just because everyone is talking about weight loss doesn't mean you need to do the same.

Learning to pay attention to your body's cues may be just what you need to find balance as a Normal Human . . . NOT counting calories or cutting out every food that you love!

Consider books like *Intuitive Eating* by Evelyn Tribole and Elyse Resch and just getting reacquainted with your body and its natural way of regulating these things! Simply put, intuitive eating focuses on listening to your body when it comes to things like hunger cues and fullness levels, and encourages focusing on your health and happiness instead of just weight.

APPENDIX D: OUTTAKES

You're about to find out that your Normal Human life will present all kinds of quirky little unexpected changes. Some will be good, some will be painful, but it's all part of the adventure. A couple of my personal highlights:

From the blog . . .

Got my hurr did

This is a random post with a random subject, but it goes to show you that sports affect about 92 percent of your life and daily choices (this is not based on statistical findings but rather my own rough estimate).

I got my hair cut today, and for the first time ever I didn't have to think about how my haircut would "work" with soccer. I tend to get bored with my hair very quickly, so I'm always open to a new color, cut or style. However, as an athlete there are many aspects of your haircut that you have to keep in mind:

Can it fit back into a ponytail? If not, can I contain the rest of it with bobby pins and/or headbands? If I use these methods, how likely am I to puncture my skull if I fall? Is it long enough to braid? Will the braid whip me in the eyeball and cause temporary blindness? What length will provide me the optimal messy bun? Should I dye it during preseason considering I'm going to be taking roughly

2.5 showers/day? How quickly would I regret it if I went the maximum convenience route and just shaved my head?

See?! There are all kinds of factors that go into a simple visit to the salon! So today, in my Normal Humanness, I threw all my hair care out the window.

Layers? Yep! Bangs? Why not! Length? Doesn't faze me.

Crazy hair don't care.

***

Have I mentioned my knees are in bad shape? Support group anyone?

From the blog . . .

I'm too young for this

Recently I traveled to France to visit my sister. Now, if traveling 15 hours over an ocean doesn't make you brutally aware of how decrepit your body is, nothing will. I can't even enjoy the window seat these days. I have to sit on the aisle so that I can occasionally attempt to stretch out my knees (my knees that have diagnosed arthritis, I might point out). Sometimes, I wad up my sweatshirt to make a lumbar support for my spine. When I finally do get off the plane, my ankles are about the size of tennis balls, and my bad ankle feels like I'm coming off a fresh sprain.

Herein lies the problem with college athletics. As a 22-year-old former athlete, I just used the words arthritis, lumbar support, bad ankles, and knees in the matter of a few sentences. And I've hardly had any serious injuries! Aside from plenty of ankle sprains and one bad shoulder sprain, I graduated without much to complain about injury-wise. So I can only imagine how people who suffered, say, ACL injuries feel.

Unfortunately, I don't think there's a (nonsurgical) solution for this problem, although I am keeping my fingers crossed for some groundbreaking medical advances. Competing in sports at the collegiate or professional level is going to take a toll on your body.

I do think they should warn us though. Which is why I plan to start a petition to include a disclaimer on all youth league sport signups. I speculate it will go something like this:

Please note: If your child takes a liking to this sport and develops real talent for it, he/she may well require early joint replacement among other medical interventions. Please sign below to acknowledge understanding.

***

Boys, don't laugh, because you're not the only ones who like tight buns. Normal Humanness doesn't discriminate when it comes to adult-butt.

From the blog . . .

Losing my best *Asset*

As a female athlete, how many times have you heard (solicited or not) feedback on your posterior? Certainly, many soccer players have dealt with the ramifications of having some "junk in the trunk"— and despite living through the smash hit "Baby Got Back" by Sir Mix-A-Lot, many high school boys didn't share his enthusiasm for big-bottomed girls. In turn, many of us never embraced our booty, and rather, longed for the day we could "lose our butts."

I'm here to tell ya, Sir Mix-A-Lot was right. Now that I've been removed from soccer for a while, I find that I *am* losing my butt and I don't like it one bit! I've given some thought to why losing something I used to despise is now so upsetting and my conclusion is centered around two main points: One, because it's making my jeans not fit as well. Do you know how hard it is to find jeans that fit an athletic build?! Find some that fit the badonkadonk and you're stuck with enough room in your waistline to shove a small child in there too. And don't get me started on the cost of replacing 20 pairs of jeans!

Two, it truly becomes part of your identity. You'd be shocked at how quickly you can transition from an athletic build, to the dreaded "flat butt."

In conclusion, this case of Normal Humanhood teaches us a couple valuable lessons: First and foremost, never take your gluteus maximus for granted. And also, sometimes even one-hit-wonder rappers can offer very sage advice.

APPENDIX E: WORKOUT PLANS

WORKOUT PLAN 1

I, _____, do solemnly swear to follow Lauren Link's advice now that I am a Normal Human because (check all that apply):

☐ I want to keep my hot bod
☐ I want to impress my former teammates and/or make them jealous
☐ I'm an athlete, dammit
☐ Other _____

The terms of this agreement are as follows:

I select _____ to hold me accountable.

I will work out on the following days at the following times:

MON	TUE	WED	THU	FRI	SAT	SUN

(Make sure to note on which days you'll do cardio and on which you'll do strength training.)

My goal weight is: _____
My daily calorie goal is: _____

_____
Sign and date

WORKOUT PLAN 2

I, _____, do solemnly swear to follow Lauren Link's advice now that I am a Normal Human because (check all that apply):

☐ I want to keep my hot bod
☐ I want to impress my former teammates and/or make them jealous
☐ I'm an athlete, dammit
☐ Other _____

The terms of this agreement are as follows:

I select _____ to hold me accountable.

I will work out on the following days at the following times:

MON	TUE	WED	THU	FRI	SAT	SUN

(Make sure to note on which days you'll do cardio and on which you'll do strength training.)

My goal weight is: _____
My daily calorie goal is: _____

_____
Sign and date

WORKOUT PLAN 3

I, _____, do solemnly swear to follow Lauren Link's advice now that I am a Normal Human because (check all that apply):

☐ I want to keep my hot bod
☐ I want to impress my former teammates and/or make them jealous
☐ I'm an athlete, dammit
☐ Other _____

The terms of this agreement are as follows:

I select _____ to hold me accountable.

I will work out on the following days at the following times:

MON	TUE	WED	THU	FRI	SAT	SUN

(Make sure to note on which days you'll do cardio and on which you'll do strength training.)

My goal weight is: _____
My daily calorie goal is: _____

_____
Sign and date

WORKOUT PLAN 4

I, _____, do solemnly swear to follow Lauren Link's advice now that I am a Normal Human because (check all that apply):

☐ I want to keep my hot bod
☐ I want to impress my former teammates and/or make them jealous
☐ I'm an athlete, dammit
☐ Other _____

The terms of this agreement are as follows:

I select _____ to hold me accountable.

I will work out on the following days at the following times:

MON	TUE	WED	THU	FRI	SAT	SUN

(Make sure to note on which days you'll do cardio and on which you'll do strength training.)

My goal weight is: _____
My daily calorie goal is: _____

_____
Sign and date

WORKOUT PLAN 5

I, _____, do solemnly swear to follow Lauren Link's advice now that I am a Normal Human because (check all that apply):

☐ I want to keep my hot bod
☐ I want to impress my former teammates and/or make them jealous
☐ I'm an athlete, damnit
☐ Other _____

The terms of this agreement are as follows:

I select _____ to hold me accountable.

I will work out on the following days at the following times:

MON	TUE	WED	THU	FRI	SAT	SUN

(Make sure to note on which days you'll do cardio and on which you'll do strength training.)

My goal weight is: _____
My daily calorie goal is: _____

_____
Sign and date

EXAMPLES

WORKOUT PLAN

I, _____HUGO GREYSON_____, do solemnly swear to follow Lauren Link's advice now that I am a Normal Human because (check all that apply):

☒ I want to keep my hot bod

☐ I want to impress my former teammates and/or make them jealous

☒ I'm an athlete, dammit

☐ Other _____

The terms of this agreement are as follows:

I select _____FRANK FROM THE GYM_____ to hold me accountable.

I will work out on the following days at the following times:

MON	TUE	WED	THU	FRI	SAT	SUN
CARDIO 12:30-1:30	CARDIO 12:30-1	CARDIO 12:30-1:30	CARDIO 12:30-1			GROUP TENNIS LESSON 9-11
LIFT 1:30-2	LIFT 1-2	LIFT 1:30-2	LIFT 1-2	CARDIO 12-1		

(Make sure to note which days you'll do cardio and which you'll do strength training)

My goal weight is: ___190 LBS___

My daily calorie goal is: ___2,800___

_____ 10/26
                                  Sign and date

WORKOUT PLAN

I, _Isabella Garcia_, do solemnly swear to follow Lauren Link's advice now that I am a Normal Human because (check all that apply):

☑ I want to keep my hot bod

☑ I want to impress my former teammates and/or make them jealous

☑ I'm an athlete, dammit

☑ Other _Alumni game is coming up!_

The terms of this agreement are as follows:

I select _my roommate Jessica_ to hold me accountable.

I will work out on the following days at the following times:

MON	TUE	WED	THU	FRI	SAT	SUN
60 min cardio (Zumba)	30 min strength training	60 min cardio circuit	30 min strength, 60 min yoga	30 min cardio (jogging)	10 a.m. 60 min basketball	

after work . . . .

(Make sure to note which days you'll do cardio and which you'll do strength training)

My goal weight is: _140 pounds_

My daily calorie goal is: _2,200_

Isabella Garcia 4/12/2017

Sign and date

ABOUT THE AUTHOR

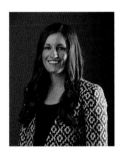

Lauren Link is a Registered Dietitian and Board-Certified Specialist in Sports Dietetics.

She is the Director of Sports Nutrition at Purdue University, where she played women's soccer in her own collegiate athletic career and was part of the 2007 Big Ten Tournament Championship team.

With a dual degree in Dietetics and Nutrition and Fitness and Health, Lauren began her professional career as a clinical dietitian with Touchpoint Support Services at St. Vincent Indianapolis, St. Vincent Frankfort, and St. Vincent Brazil—all hospitals in Indiana—before returning to her alma mater to work as a sports dietitian.

Now leading the sports nutrition program for Purdue's Division I athletes, Lauren is passionate not only about promoting optimal performance for her athletes during their time at Purdue, but also about creating lifelong habits that will help them successfully navigate the confusing world of nutrition and health when they move on.

Lauren has led multiple initiatives to this end, founding a student-athlete community garden and spearheading a program called BLAST—Boiler Life After Sport—designed to help address key components of athletes transitioning to "Normal Human" status.